TENDER TOUCH

TENDER TOUCH

by

PAUL STAERKER

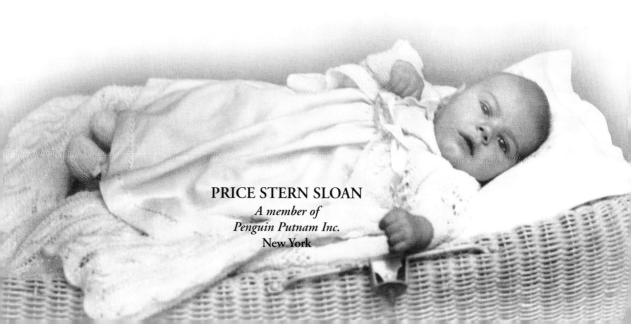

PRICE STERN SLOAN
A member of
Penguin Putnam Inc.
New York

Published by Price Stern Sloan
a member of Penguin Putnam Inc.
375 Hudson Street
New York, NY 100 14

First Price Stern Sloan edition 2000
Originally published by Media Masters Pte Ltd, Singapore
Copyright © 1999 by Paul Staerker and Media Masters Pte Ltd

An application to register this book for cataloguing
has been submitted to the Library of Congress.
ISBN 0-8431-7625-3

Editing, layout, illustrations and photography by Media Masters
Cover design and graphic art by Wendy Wong

Printed by Mui Kee Press & Co., Singapore
10 9 8 7 6 5 4 3 2 1

AUTHOR'S PREFACE

I remember being told many years ago, in my studies as a chiropractor, that a baby who was not touched, nurtured, loved or hugged could eventually die. Our lecturers told us that food and shelter might be adequate, but human touch was essential for life.

Some months ago, the lecturers' messages came back to me forcibly as I worked out at a gym where TV monitors were set up to provide visual focus while you exercised. The silent television was accompanied by the pounding beat of rhythmic music.

Suddenly, it was news time on the screen and, even without sound, I was deeply moved by what I saw. The camera panned in on a medical officer kneeling before two African boys, each about three years old. They simply stared vacantly into the distance while flies crawled around their mouths and eyes. They didn't blink. The look in their eyes was of unimaginable terror.

The man then touched their feet and hands. No reaction. He moved his hand in front of their eyes. Nothing. He tried to turn the head of one so that the child would look at him. Sunken eyes continued staring, without response, from the little boy's emaciated face, his thoughts cast somewhere far away, perhaps to the very edge of existence. The children were completely rejecting any human touch or interaction.

I fought back tears as I watched the awful effects of deprivation of human touch in children who had never experienced love, and had probably only seen the horrors of civil war.

It was at that time I decided the story of touch must be told.

Paul Staerker, DC
January, 2000
Web site: www.staerker.com

ACKNOWLEDGMENTS

Many people contribute to the writing of a book like this. Professionally, I owe much to the teachers of the National College of Chiropractic in Chicago, Illinois, where the message of touch was fundamental to my learning. In particular, I acknowledge the late Dr Joseph Janse, a brilliant teacher whose wisdom helped set me on the right path.

With the production of Tender Touch, Peter Goodall was immensely helpful with the photographic work. So, too, was cameraman, Joseph Xavier.

I thank our models: Former US champion college basketball player Cal Bruton and daughter Shakira; Helen Joyce and daughter Hayley; Kathryn Crockett and son Jordan; Sarah Draper and son Zack; Norwa binte Harun and son Mohammad; Chitra Shanmugam and daughter Devi; Michelle Saw Mei Sian and son Matthew; Alice Farroa and son Michael.

I am most grateful to my dear friend, Dr. Peter Bryner, who, as ever, has provided me with invaluable technical direction. As project co-ordinator, David Webb was a selfless editorial expert and patient overseer. A special mention goes to Catherine for her enduring support throughout this project.

And, finally, a warm thanks to all the moms, dads and babies who taught me the priceless gift of the tenderness of touch. Nobody did this better than my mother and late father, my very first teachers. To both of them I dedicate this book.

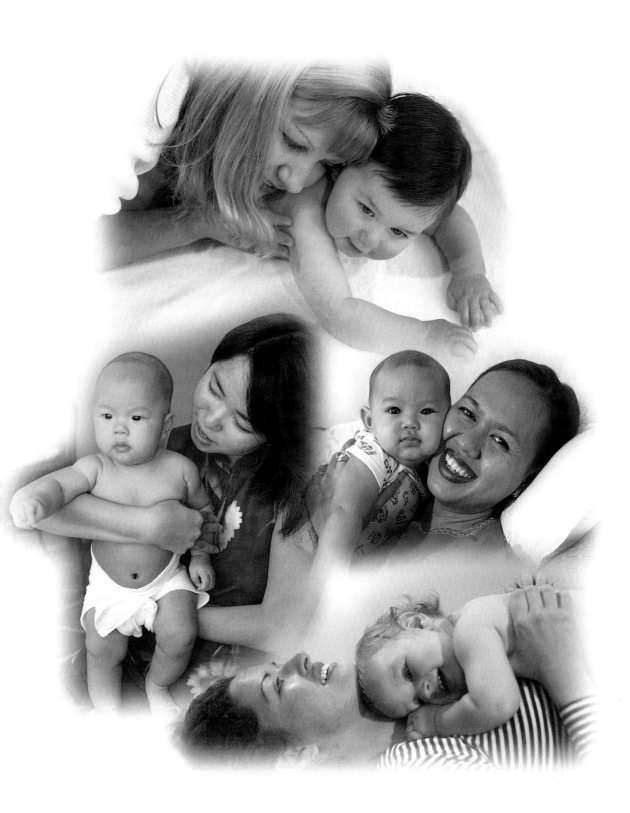

CONTENTS
Part One

Chapter 1 : The Tenderness of Touch

- The Importance of the First Touch 10
- Colic in the Newborn Baby 12
- An Early Lesson 14
- Babies Know Best 17

Chapter 2 : How and Why Your Body Reacts

- Nature or Nurture? 20
- Will There Ever Be a Computer Like This? 21
- Massage During Pregnancy 23
- Perineal Massage 25
- Massaging During Labor 25
- The Nervous System at Birth 26
- The Conductor of the Orchestra 27
- The Central Nervous System (CNS) 28
- The Afferent and Efferent Nerve Connections 29
- The Wonderful Sensorium of the Body 31
- Watch your Emotions 33
- Instinct and Intention 35

Chapter 3 : The Nature and Importance of Touch

- The First Important Study of the Nature of Touch 38
- The Benefits of a Healing Touch 39
- More Recent Studies about Touch 41
- Bonding and Emotional Development 42
- Changing the Chemistry of the Body 45
- A Touchy Subject 47
- Conveying Relaxation by Touch 49
- Touch: Emphasis on Intention 51
- Developing an Effective Habit 51

Part Two
Chapter 4 : Massage – Preparing for Action

- How It All Began 54
- Types of Massage 55

- Important Guidelines for Effective Massage 56
- When Do You Start? 65
- Finish It Slowly 66
- When NOT to Massage 67
- Get on Your Bike 68
- How Do I Practice? 68

Chapter 5 : Massage – Getting Started

- One Section at a Time 70
- STAGE ONE: Head and Spine 70
- STAGE TWO: The Lower Extremities 74
- STAGE THREE: Face, Head and Neck 78
- STAGE FOUR: Arms and Hands 82
- STAGE FIVE: Chest and Abdomen 84
- A Word About Constipation 87
- STAGE SIX: Front of the Lower Extremities 89
- Working from the Periphery towards the Heart 91
- The Homunculus 92

Chapter 6 : Understanding and Using Acupressure

- Enhancing Massage Therapy 94
- What is Acupuncture or Meridian Therapy? 95
- How Does Meridian Therapy Affect the Body? 97
- Getting Started With Acupressure 98
- Using Your Hands 98
- What is the Best Position? 99
- Points, Problems & Solutions 100
- The All-In-One Go Approach 100
- Some Particularly Beneficial Points 103
- James and the Magic Triad 106
- Lung Problems: Asthma and Upper Respiratory Tract Infections 109
- Headache and Toothache 111
- The Importance of the Hands and Feet 112
- Motion Sickness and Nausea 115
- Two Natural Tranquilizing Points 115
- Summary 117

Final Message: Good Luck, Good Health 118

Massage At A Glance 119

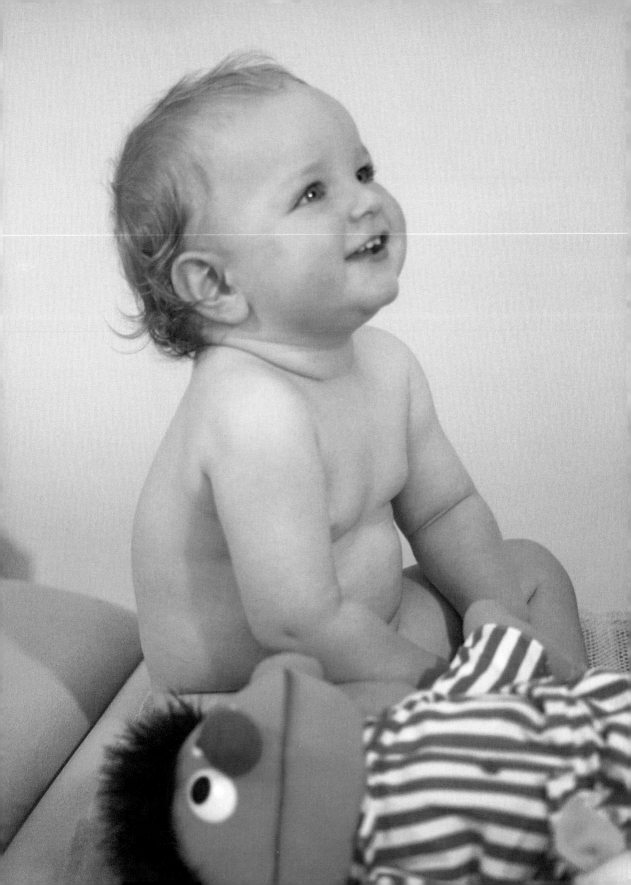

Chapter 1

The Tenderness of Touch

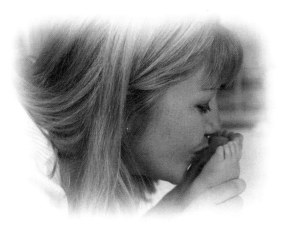

- The Importance of the First Touch

- Colic in the Newborn Baby

- An Early Lesson

- Babies Know Best

THE IMPORTANCE OF THE FIRST TOUCH

A pat on the back, a close hug, a warm hand brushed softly over a furrowed brow. Applied with caring concern, a touch can be most comforting and very supportive.

It needs no spoken word. It transmits a feeling of concern and healing. Touch totally reassures.

A mother instinctively reaches out to hold and caress her newborn child. In those precious first minutes outside the womb, the baby experiences touch, one of a human being's most important sensations. The nature of that touch can convey a calming reassurance and ensure a good start in life. However, if the mother is uptight, it can impart a feeling of tension and alarm, depending on how the touch is given. The mother's warmth, intent and feeling are transmitted to the infant through the sensation of touch. The baby's nervous system 'picks up', like a radio receiver, the vibes or feelings behind the touch.

In a sense, the newborn's nervous system is like a computer, instantly evaluating and recording the millions of bits of information which bombard its five senses. Light, sound, movement and a warm environment impact on this relatively new nervous system as it begins to analyze the nature of a strange, new world.

All in all, it can be a bit startling. Just think about it. Nine months encased in a warm, protective environment, and now it's show time in the real world!

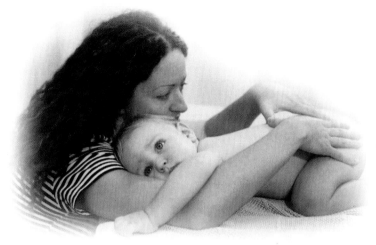

The first touch is very important to the newborn's psyche. How many of us have experienced a rather challenging birth, fetal distress, or a forceps or vacuum extraction? From a psychological viewpoint, many psychotherapists have emphasized the importance of the child's first interpretation of its life outside the womb. Was there pain, alarm, anxiety, noise? Or was it calm, warm, and welcoming? A calm and gentle delivery is considered to be very important to the optimal psychological development of the child. First impressions are the lasting ones and, if the first experience of the world (outside the womb) is of pain and distress, then there may be a lasting impression that life is difficult and a struggle.

In the physical sense, chiropractors and others have long stated that a difficult birth process can strain or damage the joints in the spine, particularly in the neck (cervical region). Chiropractors use the term *vertebral subluxation* to describe the derangement of normal joint function and alignment which can affect the spinal nerves.

Nerve tissue irritation may cause a baby to be irritable and colicky, prompting frequent crying, and distension of the abdomen and an inability to pass wind. Spinal stress created during the birthing process and the sudden change to a weight-bearing environment can generate further stress and subsequent spinal dysfunction and subluxation, seriously impairing a baby's health. We also see many examples of a baby being accidentally dropped, or picked up incorrectly without proper support for the head.

The consequent damage to the spine frequently causes pain and, sometimes, poor health. An adult can feel the pain of a subluxation, but babies cannot express such feelings of discomfort, except by crying! Colic is one of the most common symptoms associated with spinal subluxation in a baby.

COLIC IN THE NEWBORN BABY

Infantile colic is a term used to describe sudden episodes of unexplained, persistent, *full-force* crying in a thriving, well-nourished and otherwise healthy infant. It is generally believed to be a pain reaction to dysfunction of the digestive tract.

'Full-force' crying is the technical term used to describe crying which is six times more powerful than in babies without colic. A baby will also undergo *motor* unrest during a colicky episode, flexing its knees towards the abdomen, and arching its head and trunk backwards.

With normal crying, a baby stops when its basic physiological needs – such as food and warmth – are satisfied. A colicky child cries on in obvious distress and pain, despite having its physiological needs met and despite all attempts to comfort it.

Many experts believe reflux is a similar condition closely related to colic. The acidic contents of the stomach gurgle back into the esophagus, irritating its sensitive lining. In adults, this causes the classic symptoms of heartburn. In infants, the symptoms can vary from mild regurgitation to significant projectile vomiting.

About one in every five babies gets colic. It usually starts at one to four weeks of age, and is considered to be self-limiting by the time the baby reaches four months. However, those first few months can be sheer torture for the parents.

Around the world, millions of babies each day suffer long bouts of full-force crying. It is hard to imagine the stress and frustration of parents who watch helplessly as their newborn goes through hours, days and sometimes weeks of serious and obvious distress.

Lack of sleep begins to take its toll. Mum lies on the pillow, nerves on edge, waiting for the first cry. Dad is the same, walking the floor at night while the rest of the world sleeps peacefully. Parental nerves become frayed. Relationships too often are pushed to the brink. Worst-case scenarios end in the most tragic of all situations – child battering.

Parents CAN take action to alleviate the distress of a colicky child and at the same time reduce their own levels of stress. Studies show that the playing of quiet music, the dietary replacement of cow's milk with soy milk, and the use of herbal teas can be moderately effective in some cases.

More research needs to be done to establish the real cause of colic. Diet, allergies, stress in the baby, stress in the mother, mother being a smoker and other factors are all believed to contribute to the condition. Recent Danish research reported that babies with colic can have a very high incidence of spinal misalignment. The studies showed that chiropractic treatment of babies with colic resulted in resolution of colic in 94 percent of cases within a few weeks.

Clinical experience and research also show that massage of infants with colic can result in marked improvement in their condition.

AN EARLY LESSON

When I first attended Chiropractic College, I was told chiropractic care could help children of all ages. I wondered, then, how little people could have significant spinal problems. Babies, for instance, had scarcely the time or opportunity to accumulate them. It wasn't long before personal practical experience dramatically revised my views.

My eyes were opened the first time I was confronted with a screaming baby as an extern in an inner city teaching clinic of the National College of Chiropractic in Chicago, Illinois. I was a 23-year-old in the fifth and final year of the course. I had never held a baby in my life! The clinician, a huge ex-army lieutenant, grunted and said: "Fix that child and give those parents some peace!" It was an order, not a suggestion. Dr H. had never really left the army. I had the distinct impression I would be cleaning the toilets with a toothbrush that night if I didn't get immediate results!

The parents looked at me with glazed eyes. They were exhausted and at the end of their tether. Looking back, I know I was very nervous as I picked up the wriggling, screaming little bundle and promptly felt a wet and full nappy. I vowed never again to hold a baby immediately to my chest! My yellow and brown-stained 'white shirt' never did wash up properly after that.

The parents began gushing apologies, the baby kicked more and more, and I felt I might soon need a nappy change myself. Somehow my training took over. I remembered the words of several instructors – "always examine the upper cervical spine, as the cervical vertebrae can become subluxated during the birth process". So I did. As I checked, I was amazed at how tiny his little neck was, and how powerful were his arms, legs and lungs.

I felt a slight degree of tightness in the upper two vertebral segments directly under the skull. A brief history of the birth process reaffirmed my diagnosis;

forceps delivery and a prolonged and difficult labor that had strained the upper cervical spine.

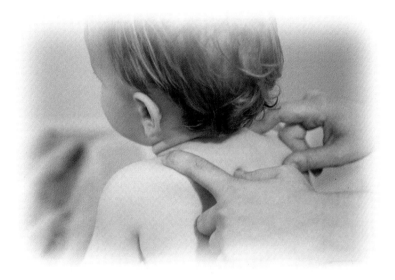

How to fix it? The same as with an adult, but with only light finger pressure. I did just that, and waited for the miracle to occur. Instead, the baby screamed even louder!

I was panic-stricken. Should I do it again? I decided to check once more. This time I found my little patient was still tight. I remembered those valuable words "Rome wasn't built in a day", and told the parents to "come back tomorrow" ("healing takes time", or so my teachers always said). I figured I would have the toilets scrubbed out by then and we could administer the second spinal adjustment.

The clinician saw the screaming baby leave, and glared at me for failing to produce a miracle. I was dejected as I drove home that night. I remember getting out my notes and books and reviewing pediatrics into the wee hours as my shirt soaked in a pail of detergent (I briefly tossed around the pros and cons of wearing a rubber apron next time, a thought I quickly abandoned).

The next day I met the couple with a head full of knowledge and a burst of enthusiasm. They were blurry eyed, but distinctly smiling. "He slept for six hours last night! The first time since he was born!" they quietly shared with me. I was ecstatic and at the same time noted that the child had managed to get more sleep than I did that night!

I noticed, appreciatively, that his nappy was clean. He was a more relaxed child for sure. I jokingly asked if they had swapped babies. I checked his neck and it was still tight, but not nearly as bad as the previous day.

I proceeded to apply gentle massage to the base of his tiny skull, using the tips of my fingers. His little eyes couldn't really see me, but he stared in my general direction with a peaceful look I will never forget. I kept up the gentle massage, letting my instinct take over. I had never done this before, but something inside me knew what to do. I felt him relax, and watched his body let go. The parents' reactions were something I will never forget. They leaned over, smiled, cooed and fussed over him. They were so amazed that he was capable of relaxing in this way. "What on earth are you doing!? Look at him, he's smiling! He loves it!" they said.

I was amazed myself. I would be lying if I said my ego wasn't swelling at a rate of knots. The thought of cleaning the toilets was rapidly fading in the light of my newfound glory. 'Wow, this stuff really works!' I thought to myself. I massaged his neck again, and the baby just relaxed into it.

As the parents departed, they beamed at Dr H. and made comments about sainthood for myself. By now, my head was dangerously swollen. The doctor smiled back, waited for them to leave, and then told me not to get too excited. "What else did you expect?" he asked, as he told me to get back to work. His remarks came as a slap in the face at the time, but, in retrospect, he really did expect nothing other than success. Indeed, what I did was nothing special. But, as the years passed, my experience with the Chicago baby would become one of my most treasured memories.

BABIES KNOW BEST

I saw the child a few more times, and he continued to settle down nicely over a two-week period. His parents also changed remarkably before my eyes. As their son improved, so their relationship deepened and healed.

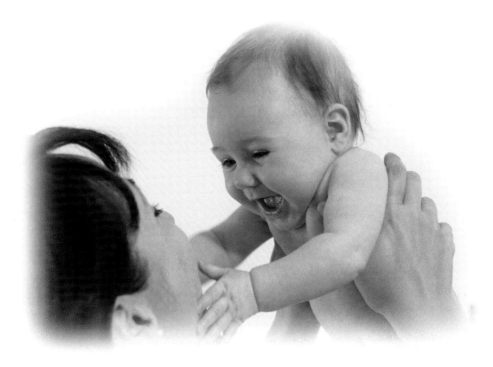

SO WHAT DID I LEARN?

- Well, babies love to be touched.

- They respond beautifully to massage applied with loving intent and skill.

- They will tell you with their body language what they like, what they don't and when they have had enough.

- The family unit itself is inextricably linked, one member to the next. Illness in one has an effect on all.

- A sick baby can influence the health of both parents, and their relationship.

- To be able to optimize the relationship of a newborn infant with its parents, through the miracle of touch, is one of the most satisfying elements in my work.

Over the years I have developed and gathered techniques gleaned from practitioners of many disciplines. I have studied books and applied what I have learned to scores of infants, and perhaps thousands of children. My goal is to share some of these techniques with you and to get you started with the basics of simple and effective baby massage. You can make a difference by using your innate calming touch. All you need is a bit of guidance along the way to help you get started on the road to improving your child's health, naturally.

Chapter 2

How and Why Your Body Reacts

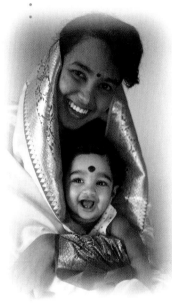

- Nature or Nurture?

- Will There Ever Be a Computer Like This?

- Massage During Pregnancy

- Perineal Massage

- Massaging During Labor

- The Nervous System at Birth

- The Conductor of the Orchestra

- The Central Nervous System (CNS)

- The Afferent and Efferent Nerve Connections

- The Wonderful Sensorium of the Body

- Watch Your Emotions

- Instinct and Intention

NATURE OR NURTURE ?

I t is no longer believed that babies come into the world with their intelligence and personality genetically pre-programmed. Neither is the opposing argument considered valid; that we arrive with a blank slate, ready to learn whatever is thrown at us and to become whatever our environment and upbringing allow. The classic argument has been between *nature* or *nurture*. In other words, does nature predetermine our potential and intelligence; or is it the nurturing we receive as children?

Actually, the truth is balanced somewhere between the two. Both our genes and our environment have an influence on what and who we become and what qualities we eventually develop and bring into adulthood. Our genetic programming (what we inherit from our parents) and our environment blend together and create a symphony to which we dance and develop our potential as human beings.

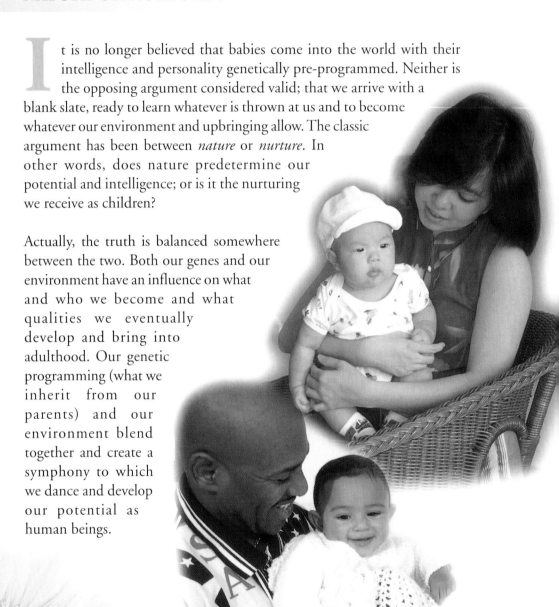

Each child has a potential for greatness, but exactly what that greatness will be is determined by experience in the first three to five years. The brain's patterns that will last can be compared to a sculptor who chisels away bits of marble, until a beautiful figure is left. The remaining figure is determined partly by the nature of the marble (the genetic material supplied by nature) and the experience created by the sculptor (the environment).

To appreciate fully how and why massage can be so profoundly beneficial to your baby's general health and well-being – and to put these special techniques into practice – you first must have a general understanding of the human nervous system. When you do, the following pages will evolve into a fascinating adventure and you will encounter one of the most gentle and rewarding experiences of your life: the closest possible bonding with your baby. It's a prediction I'd never make lightly. So, let us begin.

WILL THERE EVER BE A COMPUTER LIKE THIS?

Let us have a look at how our nervous system develops, and how our entire life revolves around its function.

Consider the first second. Sperm meets ovum. Fertilization takes place and cell division begins immediately: 1:2:4:8:16:32:64, until we finally end up with a complement of 100 trillion cells! By the third week of life a long, thin tube of nerve cells called the neural tube forms and develops at an astonishing rate of 250,000 cells a minute.

The brain and the spinal cord develop rapidly from the neural tube. This is a very precise and delicate process that can be affected by viral infections, malnutrition or substance abuse, creating abnormalities such as mental retardation, autism, schizophrenia, epilepsy and other developmental anomalies.

The genetic coding in our DNA precisely pre-programs the development of each cell and tissue in our body. Cells differentiate into buds that will become little arms and legs. Organs gradually develop from specialized clusters of cells.

At approximately three weeks, the entire process comes under the control of the nervous system. Control and regulation of every organ and each cell of the body are now under the direction of the master conductor. At six weeks of life, the brain is richly endowed with blood vessels to supply its enormous growth rate. At this stage it is almost as big as the embryo's body.

During development, the electrical activity of the brain actually changes the physical structure, and wiring of the brain. There is a huge amount of spontaneous electrical activity as neurons continually fire and 'talk' to other areas in the brain itself. This activity strengthens circuits, while others that are not used atrophy and die off. Stimulation from the outside environment enriches these connections as the connecting circuitry becomes more established and secure. All of this occurs in preparation for the immense amount of learning required when the child enters the real world and begins to assess its new surroundings.

Studies show that the fetus responds to light as early as four weeks and to sound at 24-28 weeks. This means that the little one's nervous system is in the process of evaluating and 'reading' its environment *in utero* – meaning 'within the uterus.'

Most of us have been in an apartment or hotel room where we have heard the goings-on of people in the next room. We have heard voices, laughter, parties and the occasional fight. If it is laughter – we smile. A late night party – we are frustrated as we toss and turn. An argument – we frown.

This is what it is like in the womb, where evaluation of the outside world has already begun. There, the nervous system of the fetus is continuously reacting to outside voices, music and noises.

It makes good sense, then, that the mother should begin massage of her child while she is pregnant. That's right, massaging her own tummy and humming gently can create a state of relaxation in the fetus, in utero. Self-massage during pregnancy is when the tenderness of touch is first applied.

MASSAGE DURING PREGNANCY

Although this is a book on baby massage, I must stress the need to relax the mother during pregnancy since her discomfort can easily be carried over to the baby. You can massage your abdomen yourself, but it is much better if your partner can help you with both the abdominal and lower back massage. It is easier for you, and has the added benefit of creating a stronger bond between the three of you.

We know that a fetus can sense and react to sounds outside of the mother's body. The same holds true for tactile stimulation of the mother's abdominal wall. If you simply rub your own tummy you will hear the sound created by the rubbing action. A baby in the womb hears, and feels, the vibration of the rubbing action. We need also to consider that the mother's nervous system responds to the physical stroking by relaxing and the chemical and neurological effect of this relaxation is conveyed to the fetus.

We naturally feel better if our tummy is gently rubbed when upset. Our nervous system responds to gentle stroking of the abdominal wall by relaxing and letting go. This can be also very helpful during pregnancy.

Take time each day during the last six months of your pregnancy to massage your tummy gently. Lie on your side, or sit, (lying face-up can put pressure on the placenta). Almond oil, wheatgerm oil, calendula cream or vitamin E cream/oil all help to prepare the skin and minimize the development of stretch marks. If you like, add a few drops of lavender oil to relax the musculature.

I always recommend moving in a clockwise direction (referring to someone facing you) when massaging the abdomen. Begin in the lower right quadrant (in the area of the appendix) and finish in the lower left. This follows the natural flow of the large intestine and enhances elimination. Take 5-10 minutes to massage gently all tissues of the abdomen, working from the outside to the central area around the umbilicus.

Expectant mothers can develop considerable low back pain, which may be alleviated by massaging the lower back muscles. Learn to do this in the side-lying position, working the buttock (gluteal) muscles and then the thick muscles on either side of the spine (the erector spinae muscles). It usually helps to do one side and then turn over and do the other.

PERINEAL MASSAGE

Massage of the vagina and surrounding tissues (the perineum) can help minimize the possibility of tearing during childbirth. Once again, use a fine oil and, after having a warm bath, massage the tissues around the vagina. You can use a finger (with short fingernails!) and stretch the tissues backward towards the tailbone, and then out towards the sides. The purpose is to stretch the surrounding tissues in a manner similar to what will occur during the birthing process.

Do this for five minutes a day for the last four months of your pregnancy and you will minimize the possibility of having a perineal tear and subsequent episiotomy.

MASSAGING DURING LABOR

Be ready to take your massage oils to the hospital, birthing center or the bedside (if you are giving birth at home). Explain to your midwife or doctor beforehand that you will be having your back massaged during labor and that you have been doing this during pregnancy. Ask for (or bring) some extra towels so you can wipe up any excess oils after the massage. Your partner will definitely be needed to massage your lower back during labor. This is usually best performed while lying on your side.

Of course, it is imperative to remember the need for proper exercise, rest and nutrition throughout your pregnancy. The manner in which you take care of yourself during this most important time will determine the health of your baby during childbirth and for long after.

THE NERVOUS SYSTEM AT BIRTH

At birth, our brain contains 100-billion neurons that influence, control and balance every function of the body. These neurons are supported and nourished by a network of a trillion glial cells (Greek for 'glue'). Every cell, organ and tissue is eventually supplied with, and controlled by, nervous energy carried to it by a nerve fiber. Nerve energy is basically the energy of life. Without it, tissues die.

After birth, an amazing growth spurt occurs and new nerve connections develop at an extraordinary rate. This is in response to the explosion of sensory input that the baby experiences. It is a time of fine-tuning which sees neural connections being strengthened, and some being eliminated. What is not used is lost, and vice versa.

The 100-billion neurons begin undergoing an amazing process of linking up countless connections with other neurons. They do this by spinning out fibers known as *axons*. These axons send signals that are, in turn, received by the *dendrites* (roots) of other axons. The signals are chemical reactions occurring so fast that one neuron 'talks' to thousands of others at any one time. And all this happens at a rate of several million times per second!

The axons are quite long and, in some adult nerves, can measure a meter. The growth of axons is directed by 'growth cones' that actually seek out certain proteins in the target tissues that are to be supplied by that nerve. Once found, the neural connection is made, and that tissue is now supplied with nervous energy. It is like running a telephone line from an exchange in the city, to a farmhouse thousands of miles away. The company knows the eventual destination, but cable must be laid and properly connected before that phone is fully functioning. The brain is the central exchange, and the nerves (axons) are the phone lines.

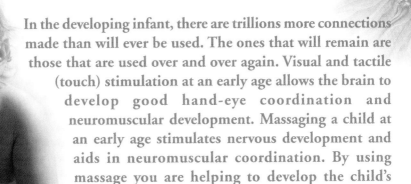

In the developing infant, there are trillions more connections made than will ever be used. The ones that will remain are those that are used over and over again. Visual and tactile (touch) stimulation at an early age allows the brain to develop good hand-eye coordination and neuromuscular development. Massaging a child at an early age stimulates nervous development and aids in neuromuscular coordination. By using massage you are helping to develop the child's nervous and muscular systems. You are also calming the child's mind and establishing a healthy mind-body image at an early age.

When a baby is born, the brain has already completed the 'wiring' for vital responses such as breathing, digestion and cardiovascular function. In the first few months outside the womb, however, there is a rush of activity as new neural connections are made. At two years of age, the baby has twice as many neural connections (synapses) as an adult!

Scientists believe this high level of nerve connections remains until 10 years of age. The brain then begins to remove those connections that are weak or rarely used. The ones that stay are those which are richly endowed by experience.

THE CONDUCTOR OF THE ORCHESTRA

The symphony of life begins on day one, the first day of conception. Initially there are a few tinkling piano notes, then chords, which gradually develop into a rhythm that flows to a regular beat. As the "melody" becomes more complex, the need for a conductor becomes apparent. With humans, the conductor takes charge around the third week of life in the womb.

The nervous system is the conductor of the orchestra, balancing all the instruments and instructing the flow, rhythm and harmony between them. A good conductor can bring a masterpiece to life.

But what if the conductor isn't doing his job properly? Then there may be disharmony, imbalance and cacophony. Notes become jangled and irritate the ears and mind of the listener. Ease becomes dis-ease.

The nervous system conducts the running of our bodies. What you ate for breakfast today was digested without a single, conscious thought. Your blood pressure and heart beat have been perfectly regulated since you awoke this morning. Your nervous system is constantly adapting to the various physical demands and experiences as you have washed, walked, driven the car and sat down to read this book. All without a conscious thought.

At this very moment your nervous system is responding to and evaluating words written months ago. Amazing. Our nervous system is the great conductor that ceaselessly conducts the orchestra of our body from birth to death.

A calm, balanced nervous system brings harmony and ease. A nervous system irritated by spinal, chemical or emotional stress experiences a loss of ease, or disease.

THE CENTRAL NERVOUS SYSTEM (CNS)

I had the great fortune of being taught at college by Dr Joseph Janse, a very influential scientist and healer and a man of diverse skills and interests. A Doctor of Chiropractic, he was also widely recognized as an author and scholar.

I remember his first talk on the wonderful sensorium of the body. He painted a marvelous picture of how the nervous system has developed over eons to allow us to interact with our environment. The central nervous system (CNS) consists of the brain and spinal cord, housed in the protective and respective casings of the skull and spine.

We have all heard that our human brain differentiates us from other living beings because of our intellect. The area of the brain that creates higher thought and awareness is known as the cerebrum, or neocortex. From the evolutionary viewpoint this is the most recent addition to the brain's functions. It is where sensations from our environment and their significance are evaluated. Here, also, is where we tag the emotional component of pain.

An older area of the brain, which we share with animals, is dedicated to more basic survival functions such as regulation of blood pressure, respiration, sexual drive and muscle tone.

THE AFFERENT AND EFFERENT NERVE CONNECTIONS

The information from our five senses travels inward towards the brain through nerves called *afferent nerves.* They transmit vital information about our environment.

Is that stove hot? Ouch! An afferent nerve coming from your fingertips tells your brain it is. Why did you instinctively jerk your finger away from the stove? Well, once notified, a nerve starting in your brain, or spinal cord, issued an outgoing series of messages to the muscles in your arm to contract and move, NOW! All this occurs for the purpose of saving your fingertip from a roasting which would cause serious harm. These outgoing action nerves are called *efferent nerves.*

So afferent nerves come in and tell us what it's like out there. Efferent messages go out to the muscles and prompt us to take action!

Nice and warm? Comfortable? How do you know? Your afferent nerves in your peripheral nervous system tell you so. You can sit a while and relax. No harm, all pleasure. Are your legs falling asleep? The sudden screech of tires! Time to move! Your afferent nerves tell you what is happening, and your efferent nerves take action and you move, away from pain, discomfort or danger towards eventual comfort and safety.

Hungry? Time to go to the toilet? Thank goodness our afferent nerves send these messages because, if they didn't, we would be in serious trouble.

We all know what happens when the nervous system is seriously damaged. Look at someone who has damaged his spinal cord, as in paraplegia. This person cannot walk because the efferent nerves are permanently damaged. The brain may want to move but the messages have no pathway to get to the muscles and make them contract.

In the normal healthy body, however, trillions of bits of information are coming in and going out at any given second. Pressure, temperature, position sense and vibration, all tell us about our environment and how our body is functioning. In response, our outgoing regulatory messages are continuously controlling our heart rate, breathing and muscle tone, thereby maintaining health and life.

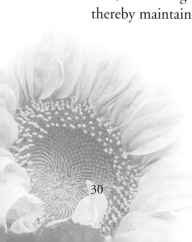

THE WONDERFUL SENSORIUM OF THE BODY

Two sections back, I made brief reference to the sensorium. I would now like to examine this aspect of human function in more detail, as it really is fundamental to the gentle, remedial measures we will be applying later in the book.

Clinically speaking, the sensorium is probably most accurately defined as the parts of the nervous system, sensory organs and skin concerned with the reception and interpretation of sensory stimuli. In effect, our complete sensory apparatus, the sensorium, has evolved over millions of years. It operates through the sensory nervous system finely developed in our skin and in the organs dedicated to smell, sound, taste and sight.

Our sensorium connects our inner being and mind to our outer world. It enables us to interact with our world and enjoy life as human beings.

As humans, we are very fond of our sensorium. We have stereo sound systems, lovely paintings to look at, scented candles, poetry, stylish clothes, and good food – you name it. We run our lives around our nervous system. And as we do so, our sensorium enables us to interact with our environment and go about our lives with the variety of stimuli surrounding us. Music, sunlight, home cooking, a lovely wine … a gentle touch.

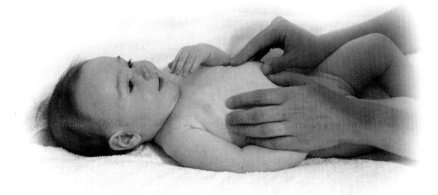

As the sensation of touch is so basic to our existence, we must pay particular attention to our skin. It is the largest organ of the body, accounting for 18 percent of our body weight and equipped with five million touch receptors in the average person. In the area under one fingertip, there are 3,000 specialized nerve endings designed to interpret temperature, pressure, vibration and the nature of the environment around us. Indeed, the skin is the organ that is dedicated to the sense of touch. Along with other functions, it also maintains our internal temperature and protects us from infection.

The skin is the outermost frontier of our body that constantly signals to the brain how we interact with our universe. It moves us towards pleasure and away from pain. It keeps us alive, and works at making the entire experience of being a human pleasurable.

We can intentionally affect the sensorium of the body in a positive way by the manner and ways in which we touch people. A smile, hug, or a hand on a troubled shoulder. The afferent nervous system of the recipient assesses the nature of the incoming messages.

It was Dr Janse who started me thinking about how the sensorium needed to be stimulated. Even in the very early stages of life, the gentle flow of the amniotic fluid over the skin of the fetus soothes and stimulates the sensorium of the developing child. Dr Janse termed it the "caress of the amniotic fluid!"

Then there are the soothing sounds and vibrations of the mother-to-be humming or softly murmuring in wonderment as she feels the first kick of the child she is carrying. She places her hands instinctively on her enlarged tummy and thus caresses her unborn child.

So the *swoosh* of the amniotic fluid is, in fact, one of the first stimuli for our sensorium. As our nervous system begins to develop in the womb, our sensorium needs regular stimulation. Ideally, this continues naturally throughout gestation, into infancy and, indeed, on through life to ensure proper development of our nervous system and ongoing harmony and health as an adult.

The wonderful sensorium of the body enables us to be human, and to stay alive long enough to enjoy it.

Meanwhile, in related activity, the brain and the immune system continually 'talk' to one another using similar pathways. This explains how the state of mind influences our overall health. The modern field of psycho-neuro-immunology focuses on how the state of our mind and the nature of our thoughts affect the function of our immune system. Indeed, through the nervous system, the entire body can be affected by the quality of our mental state. The mind/body connection has been written about and studied extensively by many scientists and researchers.

WATCH YOUR EMOTIONS

It is also known that one person's thoughts can affect the state of mind of another person. We have all experienced someone else's 'vibes.' Much study has been given to how a mother's thoughts can affect her baby's health. Thoughts create actual chemical reactions that can cause positive or negative physiological changes within our bodies. These chemicals can cross the placental barrier and have a direct effect on the fetus. Negative thoughts create negative reactions in the body. So a calm, positive frame of mind is certainly a goal which every mother should aim for during her pregnancy. It makes sense to pay close attention to the mental and physical health of the mother, since this directly affects the health of her child.

Loud rock music causes an increase in fetal limb movements, a kind of womb-like jitterbug. The heart rate can increase as a result. Soft, classical music causes a calming of the baby's movements and heart rate. Clearly the nature of the external environment can affect the baby's nervous system.

Stress behavior in babies manifests itself in many ways. Grimacing, clenching of fists, altered sleep patterns, poor soothability, irritability, fussiness and so on. A child that is calm and well exhibits a completely different pattern of behavior.

To have calm children, it is wise to start creating a calm state of mind during pregnancy. An expectant mother can achieve such an environment by watching her own health and thought patterns.

Thoughts and emotions occur as a result of, and in tandem with, the production of neuro-transmitters. Negative, aggressive thoughts, if sustained over a period of time, cause the release of neuro-transmitters and hormones that may be detrimental to our health. Prolonged stress may even lead to heart disease, cancer, diabetes, arthritis, auto-immune disorders and many other diseases.

Calm thinking, on the other hand, releases an entirely different set of *positive* neuro-transmitters and hormones.

As adults we can consciously choose the quality of our thoughts. We can alter our perspective on even the most challenging situations and thereby minimize the effects of prolonged stress on the body.

We can exercise, meditate and listen to soothing music, all with the aim of calming our body and mind.

If you feel depressed or anxious, take a long walk and breathe deeply. After an hour you will feel different. I have always told my patients you come back a different person because you have oxygenated your body and completely changed your brain's chemistry by performing prolonged aerobic exercise and allowing your mind to take in the neutral and pleasant thoughts that drift in and out as you walk.

This type of gentle exercise during pregnancy is very good for you and your unborn child.

Most people have very tight muscles indicating spinal stress. Practitioners who work with the body deal with the stress that develops in the neuromusculoskeletal system and alleviate the symptoms of such stress. The result is a lessening of tension in the nervous system and a subsequent improvement in the person's health.

This is why mothers-to-be are advised to have periodic spinal examinations during pregnancy to ensure spinal stress doesn't build up and negatively affect the body and, therefore, the unborn fetus.

It is most important that a woman be as comfortable as possible during the term of pregnancy, both for her sake and for the health of her unborn child.

INSTINCT AND INTENTION

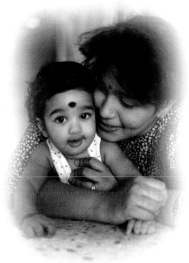

A mother instinctively knows her baby needs to be touched. Stimulation of the baby's sensorium is essential to good parenting.

But can we learn to develop touch in a way which is more effective than instinct alone? Can we learn to act with the intention of creating a positive change in our child? The answer is a resounding YES. By using touch as a healing, nurturing and calming action, we can, with intention, improve the mental and physical health of our child.

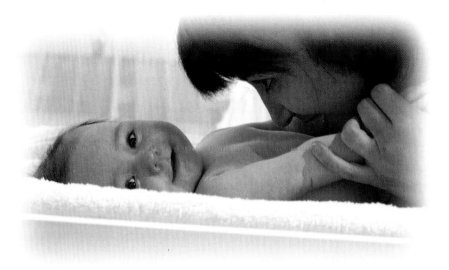

We all have a survival instinct and some of us barely do survive in this modern, fast-paced world. Others learn how to be effective in their personal lives and, with intention, go out and develop emotionally, physically, mentally and spiritually, ultimately making a difference in their lives and in the lives of others. ***Instinct*, combined with *positive intent*, is a very powerful force.**

Thus far, we have been acquainting ourselves with the general workings of the human nervous system. This is the foundation on which we will now be working as I explain the various techniques that can make a substantial difference to your child's health. My intention is to enable you to enhance positively the development of your baby's sensorium – and thereby help your child grow into a healthy and effective adult.

The purpose of this book is to examine the importance of the mind/body connection and to show how therapeutic touch, or therapeutic massage can be used as a wonderful, natural tool to enhance that connection.

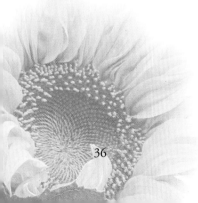

Chapter 3

The Nature and Importance of Touch

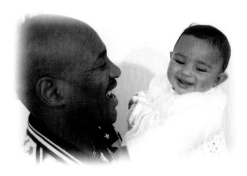

- The First Important Study of the Nature of Touch

- The Benefits of a Healing Touch

- More Recent Studies about Touch

- Bonding and Emotional Development

- Changing the Chemistry of the Body

- A Touchy Subject

- Conveying Relaxation by Touch

- Touch: Emphasis on Intention

- Developing an Effective Habit

THE FIRST IMPORTANT STUDY OF THE NATURE OF TOUCH

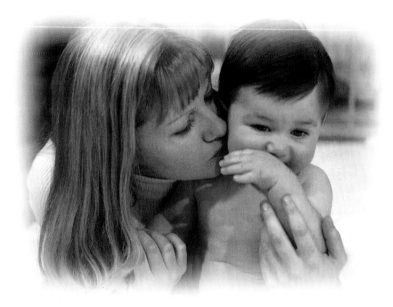

When Salimbene, a thirteenth century Italian Franciscan, sat down to write his account of the German Emperor Frederick II, he could not have known that he would be making a significant contribution to medical science. Salimbene's description of the disturbing experiments that Frederick II carried out on newborn infants stands today as the first recorded study of the importance of touch on infants. History generally characterizes Frederick II as an eccentric and erratic man known for his considerable mood swings. By today's standards he would probably be considered to be psychotic.

Salimbene wrote about one particularly cruel experiment performed at the order of the Emperor. The purpose was to determine what language children would speak if they were raised without ever hearing a spoken word. The Emperor chose a group of newborn babies and commanded they be taken from their birth mothers and placed in the care of specially appointed foster mothers and nurses. The children were fed, but there was no playing, talking, gentle touching or cuddling.

Salimbene recalls: "Bidding foster mothers and nurses to suckle, bathe and wash the children, but in no ways to prattle or speak with them, for he (Frederick) would have learned whether they would speak the Hebrew language (which had been the first) or Greek, or Latin, or Arabic or perchance the tongue of their parents of whom they had been born. But he labored in vain, for the children could not live without clapping of the hands, and gestures, and gladness of countenance and blandishments." In other words, these poor children all died before ever speaking a word.

Through this inhumane experiment he made the discovery that the need for touch (tactile stimulation) was essential for the development of the child's nervous system. Indeed, those children could not live without the stimulation of human touch.

Look Magazine reported in August 1997 that these findings were repeated most recently in Romania during the early 1990's "when thousand of infants warehoused in orphanages, some of them virtually left alone in their cribs for two years, were found to be severely impaired".

THE BENEFITS OF A HEALING TOUCH

How important is stimulation of the baby's sensorium through regular touch? Very, very important as the following study shows.

Tiffany Field, PhD, Director of the Touch Research Institute (Miami, Florida, USA), conducted a study of premature babies over a course of 10 days. The babies were massaged three times a day, 15 minutes each time. The results showed that these babies gained 47% more weight and were discharged an average of six days earlier than babies who were touched or cuddled only when fed or diapered.

It appears the weight gain was due to stimulation of the Vagus nerve that controls most functions of our gastrointestinal (GI) tract. It seems to affect insulin levels and subsequent glucose levels, leading to an overall improvement in the working of the GI tract itself. The children didn't actually eat more. They just absorbed their food more efficiently.

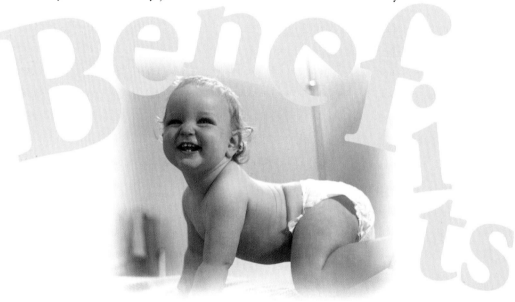

Studies show that therapeutic touch, or massage has many benefits. It:

- Alleviates depressive and anxiety symptoms;
- Reduces stress hormones like cortisol and norepinephrine. (Remember babies suffer from stress, too!);

- Reduces pain;
- Positively alters the immune system, increasing white blood cell count and enhancing immune function;
- Facilitates weight gain in premature infants;
- Increases life performance;
- Improves mood (by increasing circulating serotonin);
- Improves behavior ratings of children;
- Relieves colic, reflux and constipation;
- Relieves respiratory disorders, and helps ease chest and sinus congestion;
- Improves sleep patterns;
- Increases circulation;
- Improves elimination of waste by stimulating venous and lymphatic drainage.

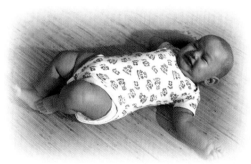

MORE RECENT STUDIES ABOUT TOUCH

Much current research confirms the many benefits of therapeutic touch and the importance of stimulation of the child's developing nervous system.

A recent study on the effect of maternal contact during infancy suggests that brain cells can degenerate and die more quickly as a direct consequence of infant neglect, impeding development of the child. During growth, certain brain cells and circuits are eliminated as neural circuits are established. The researchers found that the cell death rate doubled in animals that lacked stimulation. Interestingly, this effect was most evident in the hippocampal area of the brain, where many of our emotions are evaluated. Further studies are underway to determine the effects of this on adult physical and social development.

Numerous studies of animals and humans show that stimulation through touch and contact enriches the nervous system and, consequently, enhances general well-being. Quite the opposite occurs when there is no touching. Indeed, as some experiments indicate, even negative or painful stimulation is better than no stimulation at all.

It has also been observed that some young animals separated from their mothers for as little as 45 minutes can undergo major internal changes, including a dramatic drop in growth hormone. In such a study with animals, hormonal levels were restored better and faster by rubbing the animals' fur with a natural bristle brush than by injection with growth hormone.

A child deprived of touch will hold itself and rock back and forth. If no one will stimulate our nervous system, we will attempt to do so ourselves in the most basic way possible. The clinical picture of marasmus, where the child is literally physically and emotionally starved, sees young infants holding themselves and rocking in this manner.

BONDING AND EMOTIONAL DEVELOPMENT

We have just seen how important physical stimulation is to the physical development, and actual survival, of an infant. We now have to consider the emotional development and subsequent mental health of the child.

The nature of the bonding between a parent and a child in the first several months forms the foundation for the emotional development of the child. The quality and strength of the bonding is enhanced by both the physical and emotional warmth, caring and nurturing provided by the parents.

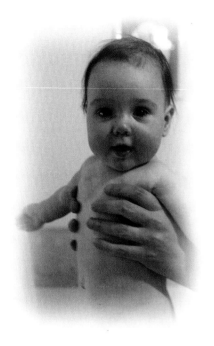

Eminent psychologist Milton Erickson stressed the importance of "a basic sense of trust" which develops when the child's core emotional and biological needs are met. What happens to us in the first few months of life sets up a pattern for the rest of our lives. Our initial interpretation of the world builds a blueprint, or foundation, on which our subsequent development is based. This is referred to as our basic existential position and determines how we actually will exist and cope in the world.

Initially, we are helpless in a physical sense. We can only cry in an attempt to communicate that we have needs to be met. As little children we have two basic needs – food and physical contact. Food satisfies our physiological needs and supplies the nutrients necessary for our physical growth and development.

Touching or 'stroking' is the fundamental act of recognition for the young child. We learn the physical outline and shape of our body by the touching we receive. 'Strokes' can also be other than physical; such as a smile, a kind word, and a warm, reassuring glance.

Ideally, someone soothes us when we are upset and crying. We calm down as we are gently stroked, by physical touch and/or soothing words. When we are happy, laughter with others is a stroke of recognition and joy, enhanced by sharing. As adults, 'back slapping' becomes a physical stroke of great importance.

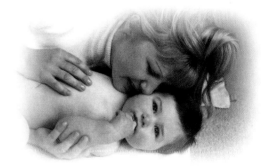

Bonding

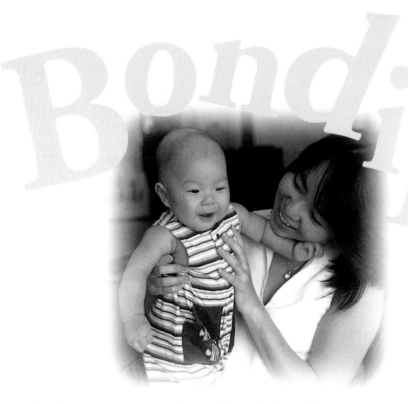

As infants, we cannot understand words that tell us we are cute or special. But we can build a solid program of who we are, based on the gentle and caring physical touch and strokes of a concerned parent. When we experience true caring and nurturing, then we decide we are special and valuable children of the world. We are safe, and loved.

Parents who are uncomfortable with touching and being close may become tense each time the child reaches for them. The message the child learns is "don't get close." Unfortunately, this message is carried with the child throughout life and it avoids intimacy in any relationship it may encounter. It is very important, therefore, that a parent realizes the importance of a tender physical touch and caring attitude when dealing with a child. It can have a long-lasting effect, touching on every relationship throughout that person's life.

The importance of one-on-one time, touching your child and providing stimulation of all of the senses, is paramount in enabling your child to develop into a capable, confident and mentally balanced adult.

There is a time-frame on all of this, and the first year is the most important. Providing positive emotional and physical support will hold a child in good stead for life. If a child is abused or neglected, however, by the age of three the marks of this neglect are almost impossible to erase.

Massage can greatly enhance the emotional and physical health of a baby and have a very positive influence on the child's development.

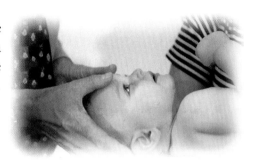

CHANGING THE CHEMISTRY OF THE BODY

Our nervous system is firing off trillions of nerve impulses every second, and each burst of neural activity is a result of a chemical reaction. These chemicals, called neuro-transmitters, are responsible for every thought and action we experience. It is essential that our neuro-transmitters are balanced, because they are vital for the state of health of our mind and body. When our body's chemistry functions as it should, we are considered to be healthy.

A child who has abnormal body chemistry through, say, drug addiction, can have extremely bizarre behavior patterns. Good health cannot exist in such a situation. But how can a baby be addicted to drugs?

I had first-hand experience of this with an infant brought me some years ago by her foster mother, Lucy (not her real name) who, for almost 30 years, had taken charge of babies being readied for adoption.

Lucy decided to look into the background of this particular child and found there was a history of substance abuse by the mother during pregnancy. This established, Lucy brought the baby girl, Sarah, to my clinic and it was immediately obvious that she was addicted to whatever drug the mother had been taking. Her screams were simply a manifestation of 'going cold turkey' or withdrawal. It was terrible to see such a tiny person writhe in such pain and discomfort as a result of chemicals transmitted across the placenta during pregnancy. An innocent and helpless little victim tormented by an unwilling addiction.

Lucy knew that her own normal children calmed down after having gentle spinal manipulation and soft tissue massage, and thought we might be able to help Sarah.

During the first two weeks of treatment she became more relaxed and attentive. She began to respond to Lucy's loving touch, whereas previously she was a mass of wriggling muscle and tears, completely detached from any effort to soothe her stressed little psyche. Within one month she was calm and feeding and sleeping normally.

I believe that by stimulating the nervous system with your hands you can help the body heal naturally through the release of endorphins and other neuropeptides produced naturally in our body. The 'pharmacy within' knows what chemicals are needed to control perfectly every function of our body. In perfect balance, in perfect time, with no conscious thought.

My experience with young Sarah clearly demonstrated how therapeutic massage and manipulation can be the most potent form of medicine available. There is certainly growing awareness that the body has the ability to heal itself, and that mustering all of its innate natural forces can be infinitely better than overloading a baby's system with foreign substances and medications which may further complicate the issue.

This is not to say therapeutic drugs don't have their rightful place in certain circumstances. Indeed, the ideal is for health care practitioners to combine their knowledge and skills and better communicate with one another for the benefit of the most important person in the team, the patient.

Altogether we treated 10 babies brought in by Lucy, and quite a few more from other parents and carers. Most of these little people had problems relating to their mothers' substance abuse. Almost all of them responded well, some better than others. I later had the rewarding experience of seeing a photo of Sarah, by then aged 12 years. She looked so bright and alive, with eyes that said volumes. Her rough start in life was made easier and brighter by the loving support of an angel called Lucy, and by the tenderness and healing of human touch.

A TOUCHY SUBJECT

I practiced in Italy for three years when I graduated. I was taken immediately by the warm way Italian families would hug and touch each other. Constantly, regularly, and not just with children.

I would watch young people walk in the piazza on Sundays dressed in their finest clothes. Men could walk with men, arms around each other's shoulders, and women with women linked arm in arm. There was no shame in people showing warmth and affection for each other. It had nothing to do with sexual feelings, just an openness to touch and physical contact.

Americans live in a "non-tactile society" as opposed to many other countries. Psychologist Sidney Jourard looked at casual touch patterns around the world and found the highest rate in Puerto Rico (180 times per hour) and the lowest in the US (twice per hour). French parents touch their children three times more frequently than do Americans.

Some researchers believe this lack of touch can lead to a higher degree of violence in adults. People who are touched more are less violent. It was interesting to see that the Italian culture, generally, was much less violent than the American culture. I lived in several large cities in America, where I had to be very aware of where I went. In Italy I never once got into a tight situation simply because the people seemed much less inclined to be violent or aggressive. I had that impression then, and research seems to back up now what I have always felt.

Could it be that the amount of touching Italian families share has an effect on the actual functioning of society? I believe there is a definite link that all parents should heed. American teachers are now told, for reasons of sexual harassment, "Teach, don't touch". The problem, it seems, will only get worse in time. A low-touch society can affect the emotional and physical well-being of its young people and eventually the social well-being of its adults.

Much research has been done on the effects of growing up in a warm family that cuddles its members on a regular basis. Children who have experienced regular, calming touch come to accept it as normal and necessary. They are comfortable with their bodies and value the importance of physical tenderness. The psychological benefits of such an upbringing enables a child to grow into a mentally and emotionally balanced adult.

So you, as a parent, can help your child develop in a positive way using the calming effect of massage and touch. After all, the depth of our human experience depends on the quality of the interactive experiences we develop.

CONVEYING RELAXATION BY TOUCH

Wouldn't it be wonderful if a mother could teach a child to relax and to be calm simply by learning to touch the child in a certain way? Touching in a way intended to soothe and heal. The intention of transmitting a calm, healing energy which serves to center a child in this rather frantic world.

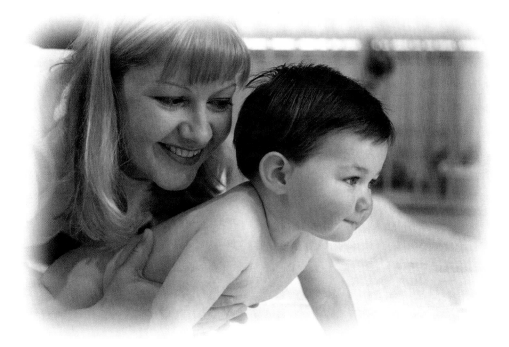

Remember that touching stimulates and helps develop our central nervous system. This is why a child needs cuddly toys and warm blankets that stimulate the skin's receptors. Touching the child stimulates the proprioceptors (Latin for "one's own sensors") and helps develop body awareness. Relaxation of the entire system occurs when the parent massages the baby with the intent of relaxing the child.

A sore shoulder, we rub it. Distressed, we wring our hands together. When suffering from a headache or feeling stressed, we put our head in our hands and rub our temples. We instinctively know massage and touch are essential in moderating our existence.

A study I saw on television many years ago still stays in my mind. At Purdue University, psychologists assessed students' perceptions of their experience in the university library. They were asked, when outside, to answer several questions about their experience that day. Was the lighting adequate and temperature comfortable? Was it quiet enough, and were the staff friendly and helpful? Was it, overall, a positive experience?

Half of the students received a different form of treatment from the checkout librarians. These students, when being handed their library cards and books, were lightly brushed by the hand of the librarian. The other half were checked out in exactly the same way, but they were not touched in the process.

They were then asked if the librarian smiled, which she hadn't with any of the students. However, the students who were touched mostly reported her as friendly and smiling. They recorded a significantly higher satisfaction with the library on that day compared to those who weren't touched.

Diane Aikerman, in her book *A Natural History of the Senses*, reports that in an experiment in two restaurants in Oxford, Mississippi, waitresses were tipped higher "if they lightly and unobtrusively touched diners on the hand or shoulder." We clearly value touch, even if it occurs on a sub-conscious level. It is an instinctive and extremely important part of our lives.

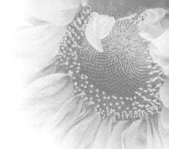

TOUCH: EMPHASIS ON INTENTION

Some people are naturals. They have a natural talent for music, poetry, sport and so on. But I very often hear comments like "I asked my husband to rub my shoulders, but he is so hopeless and clumsy! He is afraid he'll hurt me or break something!"

Clearly, there are many of us who feel we aren't 'naturals' when it comes to touch. We just don't 'have it'. This is more a belief than a truism. I can if I believe I can, and vice versa.

None of us has ever said, "I'm not a natural at walking – or eating – or breathing – or sleeping!" The need for touch is so elementary to each of us; we instinctively know that it is natural, and it feels good. It is natural for us to be able to touch another person, in the same manner in which we like to be touched.

But, I must re-emphasize; it is the *intention* of the person giving the massage that is so important. A person who intends to help and calm, and who doesn't know massage, will be of more benefit than the person who is good with her hands but is stressed or doesn't really want to help.

So, the *desire* to help and soothe is half the battle.

DEVELOPING AN EFFECTIVE HABIT

One of America's top management experts, Stephen Covey, talks about the three aspects of any habit:
1. Desire: the 'Want to'
2. Skill: the 'How to'
3. Knowledge: the 'Why' you do something

All parents *want* to help their child, and therefore have the *desire*. This book is intended to provide the knowledge (*why* massage is important) and the basic skill (*how* you go about it).

All it takes is practice and experience. Eventually it becomes second nature.

I have seen students with a strong love for what they were learning, but with relatively poor motor coordination. Their desire was so strong that they were driven to practice their art until they eventually mastered their skills to become master practitioners. I have also seen people with excellent motor skills who naturally absorb and master the physical skills necessary in clinical practice. But some of these people had a low desire to help and heal – and they became mediocre in their field.

If you need emergency surgery there would be no person alive who would want to help you more than your mother. Her *desire* to help you would be immense. But, unless she was a surgeon, her *skill* and *knowledge* would be inadequate to do the job. The mix of desire, skill and experience is a very powerful combination that forms the basis for a strong habit.

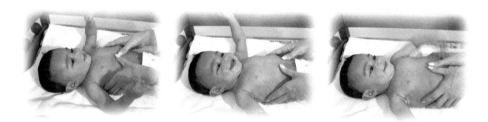

My point is, anyone can learn basic massage skills which can be developed with practice and experience. Combine this with the desire to help and you can be of immense benefit in helping your child grow into a healthy and effective adult.

Chapter 4

Massage – Preparing for Action

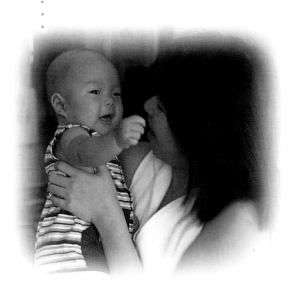

- How It All Began
- Types Of Massage
- Important Guidelines For Effective Massage
- When Do You Start?
- Finish It Slowly
- When NOT To Massage
- Get On Your Bike
- How Do I Practice?

HOW IT ALL BEGAN

The origins of therapeutic massage go back a long time and cover a vast area of our planet.

The word 'massage' comes originally from an Arabic word meaning 'to stroke'. The Portuguese word, *amassar*, means 'to knead'. Historical records and inscriptions record the use of therapeutic stroking or massage in Asia more than 3,000 years ago.

For thousands of years the cultures of the Pacific islands, India, Egypt, China, Persia, Greece, and Rome have emphasized the importance of therapeutic massage in caring for the human body and mind.

The Romans stressed the need for 'a sound mind in a sound body'. Hippocrates, the father of modern medicine, and other early Greek healers and physicians indicated the importance of manipulation of the spine and joints of the body. Hippocrates wrote: "The physician must be experienced in many things, but most assuredly in rubbing."

Over the centuries, in Europe, there have been families skilled in the art of 'bone-setting', which was the foundation for the modern science of spinal/joint manipulation. This skill was handed down from father to son, and most towns or regions had men and women who were skilled in manual therapy and massage.

Early North American chiropractic colleges taught that joint and soft tissue manipulation was helpful in treating many disorders other than back pain. Therapeutic massage was an

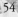

important part of the basic curricula in many schools. People have intuitively known, for thousands of years, that rubbing or stroking the body in certain ways can improve mental and physical health and well-being.

The first few years of my course were packed with the basic sciences including physiology, anatomy and biochemistry. The first 'hands-on' course was palpation of the human body, followed by soft-tissue therapy. This is where we learned the fundamentals of therapeutic massage and the importance of treating the soft tissues of the body.

In the mid-Seventies, you would have been hard pressed to find a masseur in North America. Things have changed. Therapeutic massage has taken a foothold in modern health care. Massage therapists regularly attend workplaces to relieve the stresses and strains of office workers. Many government departments in the USA offer this service to their employees.

Many people are studying massage at night school and weekend courses with the aim of helping friends and family to improve their health. It has been said that "massage is medicine." A *natural* form of medicine anyone can learn to administer.

TYPES OF MASSAGE

Just as food has its varieties and styles – Greek, Italian, Indian and so on, – so, too, does massage. There are deep forms of therapeutic massage such as trigger point therapy and transverse friction. These are generally reserved for muscle/tendon problems and rehabilitative therapy (myofascial therapy).

Some of the basic techniques of massage include:
- *Effleurage,* light stroking of the skin
- *Pettrisage,* a more firm rolling of the underlying subcutaneous tissues (just beneath the skin) and fascia

- *Tapotement,* a scissors-like tapping/striking of the tissues
- *Lymphatic drainage,* aimed at improving the flow of lymphatic fluid

These are generally lighter techniques aimed at relaxing the mind/body, enhancing lymphatic drainage, improving immune function and promoting a sense of well-being. Massaging a baby, or young child, requires using the lighter forms of massage.

Effleurage is the common technique used mostly with babies, consisting of light, repetitive strokes. These are the relaxing strokes that are usually the beginning and finishing movements in any massage.

You can certainly use a variety of techniques, but we will concentrate on a light touch with the occasional increase in pressure when indicated.

IMPORTANT GUIDELINES FOR EFFECTIVE MASSAGE

Now, we come to the all-important business of actually massaging your child. The sections which follow cover the practical aspects of how, when and where you should go about it, so that both you and your baby enjoy the experience and gain maximum benefit.

Remember that **technique is very important.** Improper technique can be ineffective, but it also can irritate the body. Some people use the term "toxic touch" to describe the negative effects of improperly applied massage which only increases tension in the person receiving it. By following these

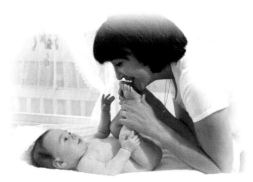

important points, however, you will readily avoid the negative effects of 'toxic touch'.

Remember that the *intention* behind the massage is extremely important! The more relaxed and centered you are, the more positive the results.

[1] Create the right mood and setting

- The first most important aspect of baby massage is to choose a room with a pleasant atmosphere, and then use that room each time. Often it will be the baby's room, which has already been decorated with mobiles and colors which are relaxing and pleasing to the eye. Have a special soft blanket ready, and use it each time. Your baby will begin to associate the feel, sounds and smells of the room with the wonderful and soothing experience of being massaged. Each time you bring the baby in and put him on the special massage blanket, his little brain will 'anchor', or associate, with the past pleasurable experience, and the entire relaxation process will begin before you even start the massage. It is like when we smell our favorite meal being cooked – our mouth waters and we anticipate the wonderful experience of eating before we even see the food!

- Avoid harsh lighting. Use soft, indirect light. Natural filtered light is excellent.

- Routine can be important. Try and find a time of day that suits your lifestyle. It may be when everyone has left the house and the chores are done (are they ever done?!). Attempt to massage at that time so your baby relaxes into the routine. Immediately after a bath or between feeds is a good time to massage.

- Keep a clock radio and other electric appliances at least two meters away from the baby. People can be very sensitive to electromagnetic radiation (EMR) which may cause tension and stress. (Much is being discovered about the negative and harmful effects of EMR on human beings. The jury is still out on this, but clinical evidence indicates it would be wise to keep clear of EMR fields, especially in the bedroom.)

- Make sure the room is warm and comfortable, and that there are no drafts blowing over your child. Have an extra blanket ready because body temperature drops as a person relaxes during massage and you need to cover the areas you are not working on.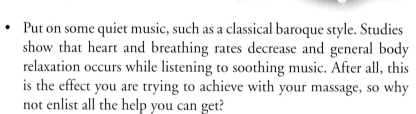

- Put on some quiet music, such as a classical baroque style. Studies show that heart and breathing rates decrease and general body relaxation occurs while listening to soothing music. After all, this is the effect you are trying to achieve with your massage, so why not enlist all the help you can get?

- Use a bench set at a comfortable height. Ensure you aren't bending over improperly and straining your back (it happens so often!).

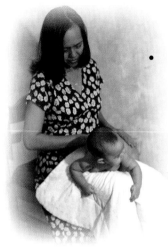

- Sometimes baby massage is done with the infant placed over your thighs, while you are seated. In this case, make sure you sit on a chair with a proper back support (a lumbar cushion helps). Remember that for you to be effective *you* must be comfortable and therefore avoid bending in ways that could injure your spine. I have seen people with a knee problem give a massage on a floor. They were then unable to get up because they damaged their knee as a result of excessive strain placed on the joint during prolonged kneeling.

[2] Other children

Many times your baby's siblings will be fascinated by the process of massage. It is wise to include them in the process. They will 'pick up' the calm nature of the moment, and usually slow down and relax themselves. If so, involve them in the actual process of perhaps massaging a foot, or a hand. You'll be amazed how many children have an innate ability to massage in a very effective way. However, if they cannot slow down, then it is best to arrange for them to be out of the room while you massage your baby. Remember, your purpose is to relax your child, and that is the major consideration.

Do involve your spouse in the process! This is extremely important in the bonding process of bringing a family closer together. Little by little, the clumsiest or most hesitant person will get the knack of massaging a baby.

[3] Do NO harm!

Health professionals all learn the first rule of medicine: Do no harm. This applies to baby massage also, and involves awareness on the part of the person giving the massage. When it comes to any form of manual therapy, always monitor the person's response. With a baby, look at the eyes. Watch facial expressions. Feel the tension in the body. As you press, does the baby pull away? If all is going well the eyes and face relax, along with the body.

If the child tenses, simply ease off the pressure and use light, soothing strokes. By following this basic rule you cannot hurt a child.

How much pressure do you use? The amount of pressure you can withstand on your closed eyelid is a safe guide; it ensures that you won't hurt your child. (Make sure you don't wear contact lenses when you do this test on yourself!)

[4] Warm, smooth hands

Your hands should be warm. If not, then rub them together briskly or hold them under running warm water and then towel dry. Make sure your nails are trimmed because a slight, quick move of the hand can scratch or irritate. Use a good hand lotion regularly to soften any rough areas around the cuticles or palms of the hands. This certainly applies to men who are manual workers. A child will note the marked difference between mom's and dad's touch, especially if the father's hands are roughened by manual work. A bit of hand cream goes a long way.

[5] Smooth rhythm

Rapid, light stroking can be annoying. Calm your mind, if you are tense, by breathing deeply and slowly. As you breathe out, think the word 'RELAX'. Breathe in, and out, over and over. Slowly, relaxing more with each breath.

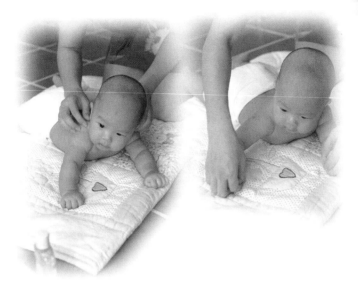

Flow nicely from one area to another. Don't stop and take your hands away at any time. Maintain contact. It can be quite startling for a person who is in a deep, relaxed state suddenly to feel a lack of contact.

As you relax your stroking, you will find a natural, smooth rhythm. You will instinctively tune into the pressure and rhythm suitable to the baby. What goes on in the mind, comes out in the body. Relax your mind, and relaxation will come through your hands.

[6] To oil or not to oil?

Some studies show that infants demonstrate stress behaviors (eg. grimacing and clenched fists) and lower cortisol levels (stress hormones) following massage with oil.

A good quality lotion or oil will lubricate the skin and enable you to perform an effective, soothing massage. As far as oil is concerned, you can use a good quality baby oil or a cold-pressed seed or vegetable oil (such as grapeseed, almond or olive oil). I would recommend using only a small amount of lotion/oil on the face, and none on the hair. Use it sparingly and make sure you warm it in your hands first (oil can be warmed up on the stove in a pan of water first).

Also, remember that some people are allergic to certain oils or lotions. If you are concerned, or if your child has a tendency towards allergies, rub a small amount onto the undersurface of your baby's forearm and leave overnight. Reddening or irritation would indicate an allergic reaction. If no reaction occurs, you can safely use that particular oil/lotion. If irritation develops at any time, try another type of oil or lotion.

Massage using talcum powder is also very popular with physical therapists in Europe. If you are powdering your baby, you can do a 'dry' powder massage at the same time using a good quality baby powder or cornstarch powder. This can also be used when there is sensitivity to oil or lotion.

[7]   For how long should I massage?

A good rule to follow is: If a baby blows its top, stop.

For newborn or premature babies, about 5-10 minutes. For others, 15-30 minutes is fine. If the child starts to get a bit restless, you know it is over. Don't feel you have to go over all the parts of the body to complete a good massage. Sometimes just doing feet and hands is plenty.

In the case of indigestion, for example, light stroking on the abdomen (shown later on in the book) and massage between the shoulder blades is often sufficient. If the baby is agitated and you get a good response in 10 minutes, then you don't have to drag through the next 20 minutes just to complete the body. Sometimes, less is more.

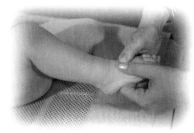

If you have only limited time, opt for a short massage of the feet. You could also do the hands, and perhaps the ears. A short session on either one or all of these areas can have a powerful impact on the body because of the cluster of reflex and acupuncture points concentrated in the hands, feet and ears.

Consider also the impact of a short rub on the spinal muscles running from the base of the spine to the back of the skull, on either side of the spine. A five-minute massage here will often soothe an irritable or colicky child.

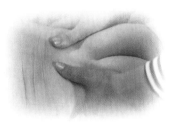

Many people in our society skip massage and exercise because they feel they need a huge chunk of time to do the job properly. The truth is, a short session is much better than no session.

[8] Which part of my hands do I use?

You can use the following parts of your hands:

- Flat palm, using *effluerage* which is a stroking motion. We know this motion naturally, as each of us who attempt massage instinctively know that we should lightly stroke an area using the action of *effluerage*.
- Flat fingertips, or finger pads, particularly good for a baby because the fingertips are so small! Small circular movements can be used in areas that feel tight. Or you can use your fingertips to glide over the back or shoulders.

- Thumb and fingers, creating a rolling effect.
- Thumb and first finger, using a pincer effect.
- Holding thumb and first finger open, in a 'V' grip. Very good for gliding up a leg or arm.
- Curling fingers around a limb and squeezing between thumbs and fingers – the 'O' grip.
- Use both hands in the 'wringing towel' technique on the arms and legs.

The age and size of the baby determine whether you use one finger, two, or a flat hand contact. Obviously the older and bigger the child, the more of your hand you may need to use. A six-week old baby may require the use of one or two fingers during the leg or arm massage, whereas an older child may need a broader contact such as an open 'V' grip to cover more area as you sweep up a limb.

Remember the point I made earlier; try never to take your hands off the baby. If you need to reach for the oil, leave one hand lightly resting somewhere on the body.

Simply by placing your hand on a person you can transfer a feeling of calm and well-being. It is important to be aware that when you touch you transmit energy. So make sure you are calm and clear about what you are doing when you touch your child.

[9] Soothe as you move

The idea, or intention, behind your approach is to "talk to" gently and interact with a baby's nervous system. The primary message to impart is that the world is safe, that touching is gentle and soothing and that you care.

Using this approach, you can just do one part of the body and be extremely effective. The feet and hands, for example, are so richly supplied by sensory epicritic (light touch) nerve endings and have such a huge representation on a brain surface that a 10-minute session can have a remarkable effect on the whole body.

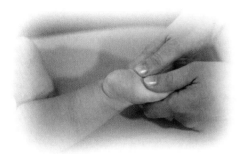

Foot reflexology, (see Chapter 5, page 76) a technique which treats the entire body through the feet, focuses exclusively on the feet. It takes a long time to master foot reflexology and I don't suggest you can learn it in five minutes. However, by following these techniques you can achieve excellent results after only a few minutes of basic instruction.

Go gently, soothe as you move, and you will be fine. If you are apprehensive, or wish to start slowly, just do the techniques for the hands or feet. Then watch your baby's eyes light up as you "talk to the nervous system."

WHEN DO YOU START?

It is important that you make the initial experience an enjoyable one for your baby. If the child is distressed or crying, perhaps a cuddle will do until he settles. Let him come to associate the massage time as a wonderful, relaxing experience, and not one of stress and tension.

Then relax and enjoy the entire experience! You are spending the most precious moments building a bond between the two of you. It is one of the most important things you can do to make this world a better place. Smile and 'be there' one hundred per cent!

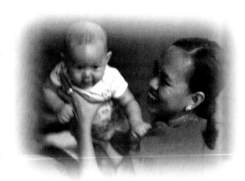

And, don't forget – keep your body and mind relaxed during the entire process!

FINISH IT SLOWLY

Remember, you have created a mood and a relaxed physiological state in your baby. It is important you gradually slow and lighten your strokes. Sudden stopping can actually startle a baby by withdrawing the almost hypnotic rhythm you have established. Slow it down, and then place your hands quietly on the baby's back or stomach for a few minutes.

If the baby's eyes are closed, then close yours too. Relax for a while, breathing deeply and slowly. This establishes a 'connection' between the two of you, and you will actually feel your energies blending.

If the baby's eyes are open and staring at you, then gently smile back, and be very quiet and still. I would suggest you savor the quiet until the baby is ready to change the mood. Remember to cover its little body to conserve body heat and avoid having muscles tense up in a shivering reflex.

At the end of a massage be sure to have the baby's clothes ready so you can easily continue with the process of dressing the child. Having to stop and run around for clothing will disrupt the mood you have so carefully created.

And it goes without saying; always have a big cuddle at the end of a massage session.

WHEN NOT TO MASSAGE

Are there any times when you should not massage someone? As with any type of therapy, that which has the ability to heal can also harm. Massage may be natural, but in certain circumstances it should be avoided. However, while full body massage may not be appropriate, you can use massage of the hands and/or feet and certainly use the various acupressure points as outlined in Chapter 6.

Conditions when massage should not be performed:

- High fever, flu-like illness, or any contagious disease.
- For 72 hours after immunization.
- Skin conditions such as rashes, dermatitis, etc.
- Inflamed joints. These may indicate a serious underlying condition. Seek an opinion from your health care practitioner.
- Bruised areas.
- Suspected fractures.
- Areas of acute inflammation (insect bites, sunburn.)
- Fresh scar tissue.
- An extremely irritable or unwell child.

Can I massage the 'soft spots' on a baby's head?

A baby's skull must be soft and pliable to allow passage through the birth canal. The skull is made up of a series of separate bones with spaces in between which can be felt as soft spots.

There are usually six of these spots which are called *fontanelles*. There are two large fontanelles on the top of the head in the midline: one just above the forehead and a slightly smaller one near the back.

The smaller fontanelles are paired on either side; in the region of the temples and at the back of the skull behind the ears. All fontanelles will eventually close up as the bones grow and the fibrous tissues ossify. This process may take anywhere from four months to three or four years!

It can be quite alarming the first time one feels the soft, yielding nature of a fontanelle. You can also see the pulse there if you look closely.

But don't be scared. Careful massage over these areas is fine. Each fontanelle is covered by a very tough protective membrane, which can withstand a relaxed and gentle pressure. Remember to use the pods of your un-oiled fingers, taking care that you avoid touching your baby's head with your nails.

GET ON YOUR BIKE

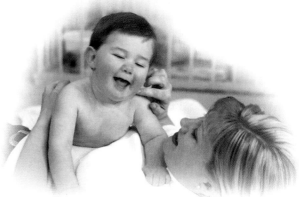

Many things have been compared to riding a bicycle. Initially it is all concentration and effort. Eventually it becomes second nature. The same holds true for massage.

In the beginning you watch your baby's reactions and, when you see a calm, relaxed response, you are on the right track. Remember, the pressure, technique and rhythm that you use are very important. Learn what your baby likes and do it again next time.

HOW DO I PRACTICE?

Just get started. Don't wait until you are good or excellent. Just start, and follow these guidelines. Your instincts will take over and, by watching the response of your child, you will soon catch on to what works best. It will become second nature to you – sooner than you think.

Chapter 5

Massage – Getting Started

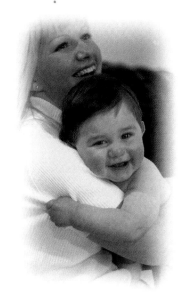

- One Section at a Time

- STAGE ONE:
  - Head and Spine

- STAGE TWO:
  - The Lower Extremities

- STAGE THREE:
  - Face, Head and Neck

- STAGE FOUR:
  - Arms and Hands

- STAGE FIVE:
  - Chest and Abdomen
  - A Word About Constipation

- STAGE SIX:
  - Front of the Lower Extremities
  - Working from the Periphery Towards the Heart
  - The Homunculus

ONE SECTION AT A TIME

A young Indian child asked his mother: "Mother, how do you eat an elephant?" Came the answer: "One bite at a time, dear". Cheeky? Perhaps. Practical? Most certainly. Large projects are best 'chunked down' into small, manageable bits and dealt with one at a time.

I would suggest 'chunking' your baby's massage into a section-by-section approach. You methodically massage and finish each section and then move on to the next. If the baby shows signs of having had enough, then stop. You will have achieved a lot simply by completing one section.

Establish an initial routine that works for you. Then vary it as time goes on. You will soon do the entire procedure with both confidence and coordination. (Remember when you first started driving a car?)

STAGE ONE

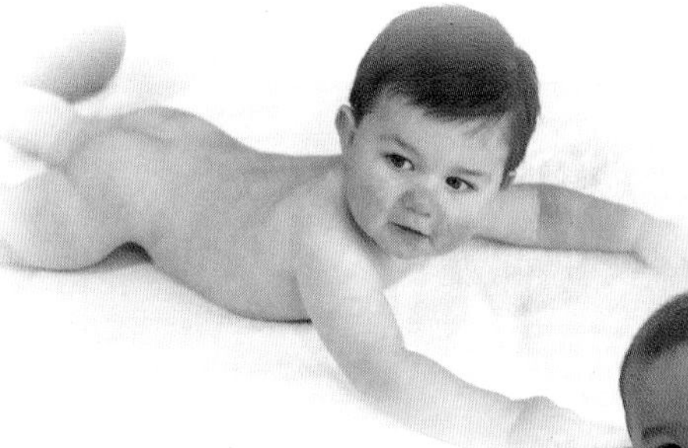

Head and Spine

**The Prone Position:
Your baby is face down
for Stages One and Two**

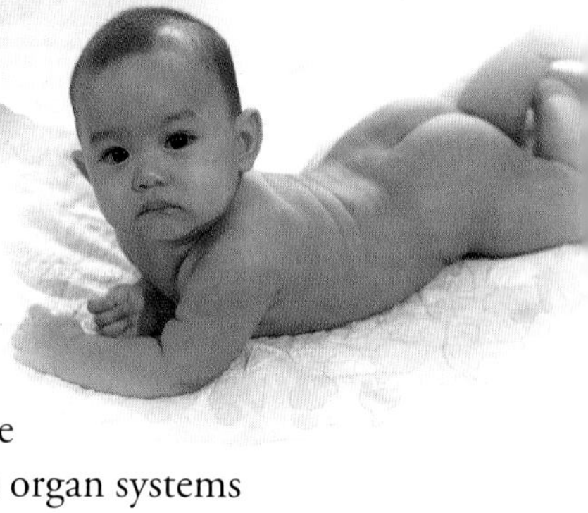

Massaging the head does wonders for relaxing the whole body. As your hands envelop the skull and gently massage the skin and underlying tissues, your baby will experience a great sense of security and warmth. This is because there are reflex points in the muscles at the base of the skull that relate to the various organ systems of the body.

Similarly, **massaging the spine** has a powerful effect on the nervous system, which in turn helps increase blood flow and relaxes the entire body. Each section of the spine affects rather specific areas of the body.

By massaging these areas, you can also influence certain conditions and illnesses. For example, the lower back for constipation, or the mid-back for asthma. A more detailed list of organs and conditions which respond beneficially to massage appears in the next chapter.

Now let's get on with our first massage. Place your baby face down (prone position) and gently stroke the following areas:

- From the top of the head, back towards the base of the skull where it joins the neck. You don't need any cream because of the hair. Light strokes are just fine using the pads of the fingers.

- From the upper neck/base of skull, sweeping down the back of the neck out onto the trapezius muscles to the tips of the shoulders, using the pads of your fingers. You could also sweep in the opposite direction from the shoulders up the neck, towards the head using your thumbs or fingers.

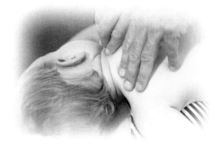

- Sweep from the center of the midback (between the shoulder blades) up towards the head, using the fingertips and flat of the hands (or thumbs), out over the trapezius muscles to the tips of the shoulders.

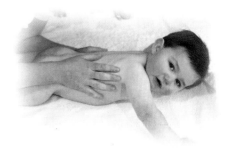

◎ Knead the trapezius muscles and shoulder joints by placing your hands gently on top of the shoulders/trapezius area with your thumbs at the back and fingers in the front.

◎ Now go to the lower back and, using your thumbs on the muscles on either side of the spine, sweep upwards to the base of the neck. You can finish each stroke by moving out again over the trapezius muscles to the tips of the shoulders. It may help to use the flat of your hands/fingers to cover the rest of the back out to the side of 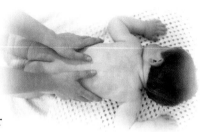 the torso. This way you are covering the entire posterior aspect of the body, which is very relaxing. Let your hands glide lightly back down the spine as you return to the small of the back with each stroke.

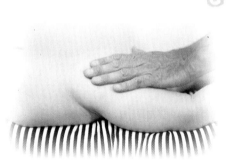

◎ Sweep the sacrum (bottom of the spine between the buttocks) and buttocks using your thumbs and/or the flat of your hands. Work from the center outwards so that your thumbs end up sweeping over the sides of the pelvis and above the hip joints. Remember to work the buttocks, but not too far up, so that you don't push on the bony pelvic crest (just below where your belt would sit).

◎ However, necessity is so often the mother of invention. So, remember that you should always be ready to adapt the massage to suit the moment. For instance, if you have trouble keeping your baby in the prone position, try the alternative, improvised buttock massage illustrated here.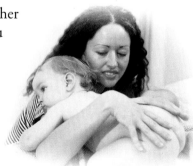

You can finish off with several light, but not ticklish, sweeping motions from the base of the skull all the way down to the sacrum/buttocks using your fingertips.

While you are undertaking Stage One, remember to turn your baby's head every so often. Approximately half the massage should be undertaken with the baby's face looking left, the other half looking right. Often there is a tendency for the child to favor one side. A conscious effort should be made to avoid this. It is far better for the baby's neuromuscular system to maintain a left-right balance by positioning the head right and left for equal periods of time.

Young Jordan and Spinal Massage

Jordan was six weeks old and suffering from severe colic and irritability. His mother and father waited each night for his crying bouts that would go on for hours and keep everyone awake. It seemed he would pick up their tension like a tiny receiving station, and off he would go with a set of lungs powerful enough to shatter glass.

He would wake for a feed and then draw his legs up in pain and the screaming would begin. It was clear his parents needed to calm him down after his feed. I taught his mother to place Jordan against her chest, face to face. If he had just fed, she would place him in this position while seated. She would then run her fingers the full length of his spine in an upward motion, massaging the muscles on either side. Then she would gently knead his buttocks and Jordan would fall asleep within five minutes. Before his mother used this approach, Jordan would scream and kick for several hours, his parents getting more and more stressed in the process. She found that he relaxed most when she concentrated on the area between his shoulders. (Note that this area affects the stomach, liver and small intestines.)

Jordan's parents were ecstatic. Now they had a technique they could use to soothe and relax their baby.

I would stress here that Dad is an integral part of the process for several reasons. Firstly, he is involved. Secondly, he can take the baby after the feed and perform the massage while Mom gets a well-deserved break. Rather than frustration, he can share a sense of fulfillment.

STAGE TWO

The Lower Extremities

Massaging the legs of an infant or child is very important. Stimulation of the nerve endings and muscles enhances neuromuscular coordination and can help the child during the stages of walking and gait development.

Also, as we will explain further on, the feet are loaded with reflex points which can impact on all areas and organs of the body. Just like grown-ups, babies love to have their feet and legs rubbed. And why not? It is simply very good for everyone at all stages of life.

Again, your baby has to be lying face down for this massage:

- Sweep the leg (anatomically the part below the knee) using the flat of your hand, thumb or finger pads, starting at the heel and working upwards to the back of the knee joint.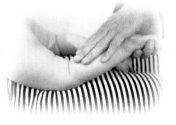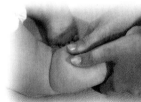

- Gently hold the knee with both hands by wrapping your fingers around the front, above and below the kneecap, thereby leaving your thumbs free to massage the tissues behind the knee. A circular motion of the thumbs works best, the emphasis being upward towards the heart. Avoid pressure on the kneecap with your fingers, which can be irritating.

Sweep up the back of the thigh from the knee to the buttocks, moving onto the buttocks and then out towards the hip joint. Use your finger pads, or the flat of your thumb.

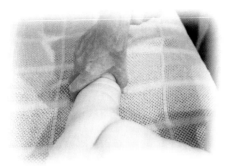 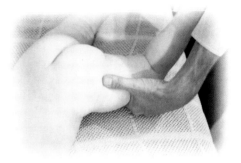

Return to the foot and work the ankle joint on the front, sides and back and then rub the heel. Work the top and bottom of the foot from the toes to the heel. Concentrate on the ball of the foot for a while. Fingertips or pads work well in this area.

You may also use your thumb, sweeping from the base of the toes/ball of foot to the heel. Or work the top and bottom of the foot simultaneously with the thumb on the sole and fingers wrapped around the top of the foot.

REFLEXOLOGY AREAS

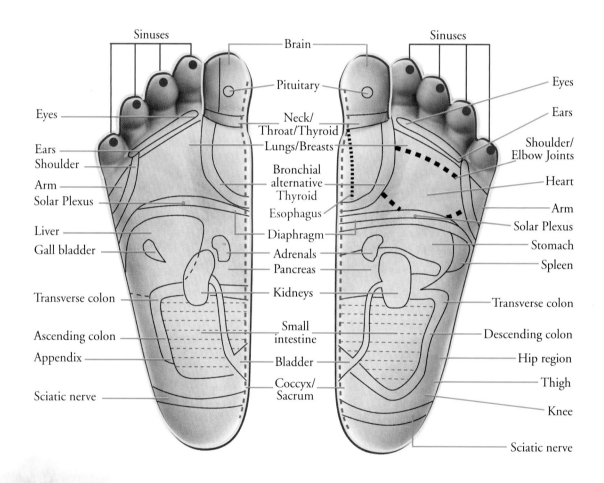

Right Foot (sole)   Left Foot (sole)

Sinuses   Brain   Sinuses

Pituitary   Eyes

Eyes   Neck/Throat/Thyroid   Ears

Ears   Lungs/Breasts   Shoulder/Elbow Joints

Shoulder   Bronchial alternative Thyroid   Heart

Arm   Esophagus   Arm

Solar Plexus   Diaphragm   Solar Plexus

Liver   Adrenals   Stomach

Gall bladder   Pancreas   Spleen

Transverse colon   Kidneys   Transverse colon

Ascending colon   Small intestine   Descending colon

Appendix   Bladder   Hip region

Sciatic nerve   Coccyx/Sacrum   Thigh

Knee

Sciatic nerve

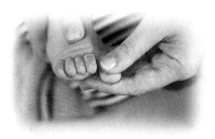

Spend a bit of time massaging the pad of each toe.

There are also many reflex areas on the bottom of the foot. Refer to the foot reflexology illustration on page 76 and note areas corresponding with any health problems your child may have. You can then work a bit more on these areas. Watch for any reaction from tenderness. This may indicate a problem that requires lighter pressure and a need to follow-up in 48 hours with further treatment.

It is also important to note that some people can have a reaction to treatment, which indicates that the body's own healing mechanism has been stimulated into action. We wouldn't expect much of a reaction in small children, whereas an adult with a chronic condition may have quite an intense reaction (such as headache, fatigue, nausea, or fever). Even a strong reaction is viewed positively, however, and treatment is altered but certainly not withdrawn.

A child with a chronic or recurring condition, such as frequent colds, or tonsillitis, may react by having a flare-up. If you have any concerns, contact your health care practitioner for reassurance and advice.

Rebecca and sweet sole music

Rebecca was a hyperactive five-month-old who just wouldn't slow down. Her problems seemed to relate to a difficult birth and, like so many children with similar experiences, she had developed a rather tense and irritable behavior pattern.

I showed her mother some foot massage techniques after noticing that Rebecca loved having her feet held. She seemed to calm down in a matter of minutes as gentle massage was applied to the soles of her feet. It was as though her feet were a miraculous dimmer switch that toned down the hyperactivity in her small body. In a matter of moments, her anxiety and tension were replaced by tranquillity. She was, of course, responding to gentle stimulation of the reflex and meridian points on the feet.

Rebecca's mother also began simple leg massage. At first she felt a bit awkward doing it. But I encouraged her to persevere and rely on her maternal instincts (Fathers, of course, have paternal instincts and they work equally well in these circumstances!) Soon she found she could calm Rebecca within five minutes just by working the feet. She would then work up the legs and, by that time, Rebecca was in seventh heaven. Her mom would hum to Rebecca as she massaged her feet and we joked that it must be the sweet 'sole' music doing the trick.

Sometime later, Rebecca's mother told me that her baby had now started making a fuss if she didn't get her regular massage! I thought that this was really a small price to pay for such a wonderful result. Rebecca's mom agreed with me most emphatically, because she realized just how beautifully her baby's nervous system responded to massage of the lower extremities.

STAGE THREE

Face, Head and Neck

The Supine Position: Your baby is face up for Stages Three to Six.

The face and cranium have a highly developed nerve supply and, consequently, a very large representation on the brain's surface (see page 91 – the Homunculus). Stimulation of the nerve endings of the head and face produces a pervasive calming effect on the entire central nervous system.

Massaging the front of the neck also aids lymphatic drainage of the tissues in the head and neck. This, in turn, may provide relief for conditions such as tonsillitis, upper respiratory tract infections and asthma. The lymph glands are an important part of our immune system and one of their major functions is to drain away waste material. But like any drainage system, the lymphatic system can become blocked or sluggish. Massage helps get it moving again.

The baby lies face up for these massage procedures. Make sure there is sufficient soft padding under the back of the head so that the child is completely relaxed and comfortable. A small rolled towel under the neck will ensure proper neck support.

When you massage the face use both hands at once, working symmetrically on either side of the head, face and neck. Each movement should be done several times.

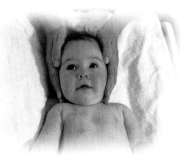

Place yourself at the baby's head with both hands in a prayer position, cradling the head with your fingers lying along the sides of the face and jaw. Apply gentle pressure with your hands alongside the baby's face. Look into your baby's eyes as you cradle the head and watch as a state of relaxation soon drifts in. This is a very safe and secure position for a baby to experience. I call this technique the 'prayer hold'.(Many therapists note that psychological trauma from a difficult birth can be dealt with by using variations of this soothing technique.)

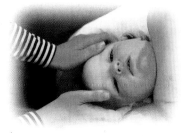

Place your thumbs at the top of the head and sweep outwards several times towards the baby's ears. Work from the center of the top of the head using the flat of the thumbs and finish just above the ears.

Use your fingertips and perform circular massage along the temples for a minute or so. Specific points in this area (the temporosphenoidal line) correspond to the major muscles and organs of the body. Massaging the temples will help relax the entire body.

Sweep the forehead using your thumbs, moving outwards from the center of the forehead to the temples.

Massage the tissue below the eye, from the nose, outwards to the cheekbones. The maxillary sinuses lie under this area and these tissues can become quite tender if the child has chronic catarrh or a bad cold. Massage here aids sinus drainage and relieves congestion.

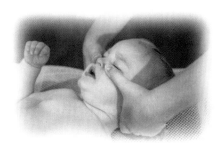

Massage the soft cheek muscles by sweeping outwards between the upper lip and nose and ending at the angle of the jaw below the ear.

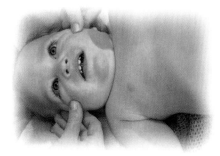

Work below the lower lip, outwards along the jaw to the area under the ear.

Sweep the tissues of the throat immediately under the jaw, moving from the center under the chin

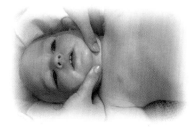

outwards to the tissues of the throat below the ear. Then stroke down the front of the neck (immediately below the ears) to the breastbone (sternum) and collarbones on both sides. You can use your finger pads, or the flat of your thumbs. Work the sides of the neck (in the front) and with several sweeps work towards the front of the neck. ***Avoid the midline directly over the windpipe.*** (Besides being uncomfortable, you can initiate a cough reflex in the area immediately above the breastbone.) All massage in the area of the front of the neck is done very gently.

Massage the ears by grasping them simultaneously between your thumb and forefinger. Using a pill-rolling motion, softly knead the entire fleshy area of the ear from the top down to the lobes. Massage the lobes for a while. A light downward pull of the lobes, followed by a 'folding' of the ear forward as if to cover the ear hole (meatus) is very soothing.

Fixing Martin's ear problem

Seven-year-old Martin had chronic glue ear. After considerable antibiotic therapy, his condition hadn't changed at all. His parents asked me if there was anything they could do to help improve his situation. I suggested that massage might be beneficial and they responded immediately and enthusiastically to the idea. I showed them how to perform massage of the neck, shoulders and cervical spine. The aim was to improve lymphatic drainage of the face, ears and throat and to stimulate circulation in these areas.

Within several months his ears improved. At the time of writing he had not had any antibiotic therapy for two years. While he did have periodic colds, they resolved quickly and did not affect his ears as before. Clearly, improving drainage and circulation of the ears and throat had increased tissue resistance and immunity. Indeed, he was a very changed boy.

Currently researchers are investigating the effectiveness of manipulative and massage therapy in the treatment of chronic otitis media and glue ear. We know that in certain cases it can be extremely effective, because nerve irritation in the upper cervical complex seems to affect circulation and tissue resistance in the upper respiratory tract, sinuses and middle ear. Cases of chronic or acute infection often show remarkable improvement in a short time with massage. In the event of infection, however, always seek the opinion of your health care practitioner. You may need to combine medical or other recommended treatment with gentle massage. Once any infection is cleared up, you can then maintain good health with regular massage as outlined.

The ear is a particularly important area in oriental medicine. As with the feet and hands, the Chinese believe every part of the body is reflected on the surface of the ear. The study of Applied Kinesiology emphasizes that massaging the ears can increase body energy. Watch your child's eyes as you work the ears. The results can be astounding.

STAGE FOUR

Arms and Hands

Massaging the upper extremities relaxes a person very quickly. Our hands are always busy; reaching, touching, and exploring. They are our link to the world as we feel our way through it. By calming our hands, we can calm our mind.

Gentle massage of the hands and the arms sends soothing messages to the brain, creating a feeling of well-being quickly.

Later we will discuss the Tsing points in acupuncture and the healing effect that simple massage of the fingers can have on the organs of our body.

For the following massage, the baby may lie face up, or even be seated. So you can do this while you are sitting and waiting to pass the time! You may use one or both hands for all of the following procedures:

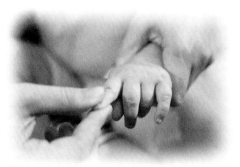

🌀 Start at the fingertips and massage each finger for a few seconds. Be aware that the Tsing points of the upper body acupuncture meridians are located on the thumb and fingertips. These points are very powerful and effective! Work each finger and thumb using your finger and thumb.

🌀 Work the palms and tops of the hands from the wrists to the fingers, using the thumbs and fingers of both hands in a pincer-like action. You can do the top (dorsum) and bottom (palmar aspect) of the hands at the same time. Use your fingers on the tops of the hands, and your thumbs on the bottom or vice versa.

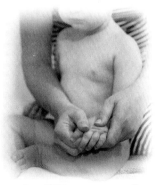

🌀 Work from the wrist up the forearm to the elbows, using gliding motions from wrist to elbow, covering all aspects front and back.

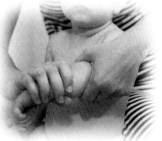

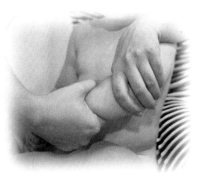

◎ Stop at the elbows for a minute and massage the fleshy area in the region in the front of the elbow joint.

◎ Massage up the arm from the elbow to the shoulder joints, working the biceps and triceps muscles.

◎ Start over again and work up from the wrist to the shoulder using an action similar to wringing out a towel (twisting hands in opposite directions). Grasp the baby's forearm between your first fingers and thumbs, thereby creating an "O" shaped ring with your hands. The idea is to improve venous return to the heart and increase lymphatic drainage.

STAGE FIVE

Chest and Abdomen

Massaging the chest loosens up and relaxes the entire rib cage, making it easier to breathe more freely and efficiently. Concentrating on the abdomen can help ease constipation, reflux or colic. You can actually feel blockages clear under your hands as you work.

However, it is important to note that massage is to be avoided when there is acute gastroenteritis or diarrhea. Likewise, if there appears to be severe abdominal discomfort, seek medical attention and do not attempt to massage. If the baby or child is in obvious pain, then avoid massage until the condition settles down. Massaging the spine may be possible, as long as the child is not too distressed.

Your baby is lying comfortably on its back. You stand or sit at its feet, looking down at the baby:

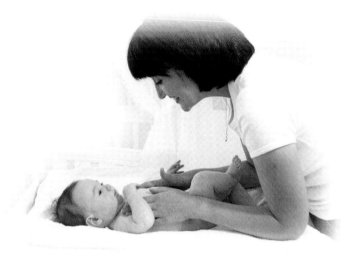

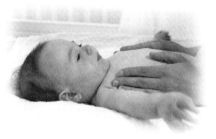 Using the flat of your hands and fingers, sweep out from the center to the sides of the chest. Remember to follow the sweep of the ribs, which run at a downward angle from the sternum.

Work the diaphragm immediately under the ribcage where the stomach begins. Coughing due to a cold or asthma will cause a tightening in this area. A lot of relief can be provided by sweeping outwards from the center to the sides along the under-margin of the ribs. Six to 12 strokes should be sufficient.

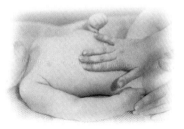

The belly, or abdominal, massage should start around the belly button (umbilicus). With newborn babies, wait until the umbilical cord has dropped off before working this area.

Work the entire colon by using your thumb or the pads of the fingers, starting in the lower right quadrant of the abdomen, where the appendix lies. Work up towards the right shoulder just below the last rib (upper right quadrant). Make three to six sweeps, depending on how the baby reacts to your touch. You then make a turn to the baby's left side, travelling across the abdomen just below the rib cage and above the umbilicus (ending in the upper left quadrant). This is the transverse colon. Once again, 6-12 strokes will do.

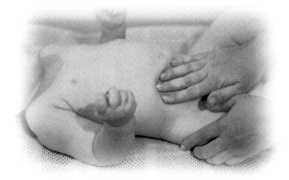

Then massage from the upper left quadrant and head 'south' (footwards) to the lower left quadrant, stopping in the abdominal tissues above the groin area.

The idea with massaging the colon is to move fecal material in a clockwise direction (facing the baby) up the ascending, across the transverse, and down the descending colon to the rectum. This is the direction of peristalsis, or normal intestinal contractions that serve to move waste material through and out of the body.

Sweep your hands over the genital area, being careful not to avoid it. Because this is a sensitive issue in societies worldwide, it can lead to us avoiding touching our own children in the most natural way. This can actually cause the child to have a negative sexual body self-image with damaging long-term effects. Be natural and gently sweep over the area, like any other part of the body.

A Word About Constipation

Babies get constipated like anyone else. A blocked bowel doesn't make a good topic for social conversation, but the truth is it bothers so many of us. Constipation causes absorption of toxic wastes into the body, leading to illness and irritability.

Inadequate water intake contributes to constipation, so make sure your child drinks plenty of water. A good water filter can remove many of the chemicals and heavy metals from tap water, making it more pleasant and healthy to drink.

A friend of mine who is a masseuse always insists that her clients have a glass of water before and after a massage. Alison will not let you get out the door without drinking at least one, and maybe two glasses. Why? Because massage stimulates circulation and the removal of waste from the body. You need to help the kidneys with plenty of water so that they can do their job of removing liquid waste.

The bowel is the same. Massaging the bowel stimulates elimination of waste from the body. Adequate water intake finishes the job. A constipated baby is an unhappy baby. Gently massage the abdomen and thereby assist the natural body function of eliminating fecal waste. Have a bottle of water nearby and let your baby sip constantly all day long. I have seen so many children 'turn around' once their bowel function and elimination had improved.

Getting Gerard moving again

Gerard was a listless 16-month-old boy who would sometimes go three to five days without moving his bowels. He had frequent colds, a noticeable lack of energy, and periods of marked irritability. His abdomen felt rigid and tense, and he pulled his legs up in pain when I palpated the area around his umbilicus.

His water intake was very low which we took steps to remedy. I began to massage his abdomen and taught his mother and father how to massage the colon correctly with the aim of getting some 'traffic flow' going in the area. They were instructed to do this for up to 5-10 minutes twice a day.

At first, Gerard didn't enjoy it at all. He reacted in a painful manner and would cry to the point where his parents were sure they were hurting him. But they persisted and, after three days, he began to have bowel movements that were quite different. Instead of his usual marble-hard 'rabbit droppings', he would fill his diapers with runny stool. I point this out because his body was naturally reacting in an intense manner and clearing months of congestion and blockage.

This persisted every day for a week, after which he started to calm down and enjoy the massage. About the same time his bowel movements normalized and he began to have a smooth motion twice a day. He responded beautifully to the application of therapeutic massage to his abdominal organs. He became calmer, and started to smile and laugh in a manner that his parents had never seen. He was a changed child.

Results such as this are not unusual. Many children respond remarkably to abdominal massage which, as with young Gerard, can make all the difference in the world.

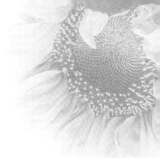

STAGE SIX

Front of the Lower Extremities

Massaging the front of the legs and thighs completes the lower extremity massage and enhances neuromuscular coordination and growth as previously stated. You must attempt to massage the front and back of the body whenever possible (ie, when the baby allows!).

Also, Tsing points are found on the toes and, when stimulated, have a far-reaching beneficial effect on the body. More about this in the next chapter.

Your baby should be lying comfortably on its back with the usual support under the neck and a rolled-up towel under the back of the knees. This allows the low back to relax completely and takes strain off the hip joints. Even a very flexible baby will find this position deeply relaxing. Remember to do each movement about 3-6 times. It may help to hold the foot with one hand and stabilize the leg while you massage with the other. (This is important if the baby tends to kick its legs around).

Sweep the front of the legs from the ankle to the knee. Cover the outer (tibialis anterior) and inner muscles by placing your thumb and forefinger around either side of the shin. Your thumb will lie against the inner aspect, with your fingers against the outer, or vice versa, depending on which hand you use. Move in a smooth stroke towards the knee.

⟳ Use the flat of your hand and fingers to sweep up the front of the thigh from the knee to the hip. Then use your fingers to massage the outer part of the thigh from the knee to the area overlying the outside of the hip.

⟳ Massage the top of the foot by holding the baby's right heel in your left hand. Use your right thumb to stroke the foot from the toes to the front of the ankle. Take a few moments to massage the tissues around the front of the ankle joint.

⟳ Gently hold each toe with your thumb and first finger. Give a soft squeeze and then a very mild pull on the toe. Very lightly stretch each toe up towards the knee. You can play "This little piggy" as you massage each toe.

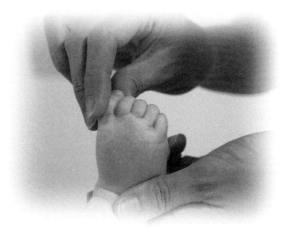

⟳ Push headward on the ball of the foot, bending it up towards the shin, while holding the back of the leg or heel in the other hand. Feel the pull in the calf muscle. Here you combine massage with stretching and this helps the entire lower leg to relax.

Now work up the lower limb from the ankle to the thigh using the "O" grip and towel-wringing technique you used on the arms.

Working from the Periphery Towards the Heart

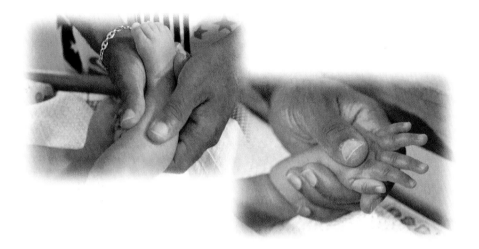

I have chosen to work from the periphery to the center of the body, or from the feet and hands towards the heart, because this is in accordance with the lymphatic and venous drainage of the body. Also, veins are thin-walled and their valves allow blood flow towards the heart only. Massaging outwards, towards the feet, is contrary to venous flow and may damage the valves in an adult, causing varicose veins.

Many therapists do the opposite in children, working down the legs and arms. I was taught, and have followed, the school of thought that respects the natural flow of lymphatic and venous blood. I feel the theory holds for young and old alike. This is particularly important in the lower extremities. It isn't a concern at all when dealing with the torso (back, chest) and abdomen.

The Homunculus

The homunculus is the "little man" mapped out on the sensory area of our brain's cortex. The nerve endings from each area of our body run up our spinal cord and then to the higher centers of our brain where we consciously interpret our world.

Note that the "little man" has unusually large hands, feet and a face. This is no accident or quirk of the artist's pen. The fact is we have a huge amount of nerve endings in our hands and feet due to the massive development of tactile and proprioceptive nerves in these areas of our body.

The homunculus is the "little man" with unusually large hands, feet and a face.

Our hands and feet are how we reach out and step forward into our world from our very first days. We grasp, feel, touch and sense our environment and a vast majority of the information about the environment comes from these parts of our body. Likewise, our face contains the highly developed senses of sight, sound, taste, smell and expression.

Our brain, therefore, needs a proportionately large area on its surface to interpret the vast amount of information that floods in from the hands, feet and face.

Massage of these areas has a very significant impact on the entire nervous system because of the 'magnification' effect as shown on our little homunculus.

Chapter 6

Taking Massage Further

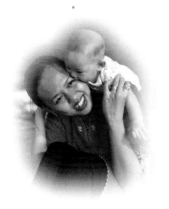

- Enhancing Massage Therapy

- What is Acupuncture, or Meridian Therapy?

- How Does Meridian Therapy Affect the Body?

- Getting Started With Acupressure

- Using Your Hands

- What is the Best Position?

- Points, Problems and Solutions
  - The All-In-One Go Approach
  - Some Particularly Beneficial Points
  - James and the Magic Triad
  - Lung Problems: Asthma and Upper Respiratory Tract Infections
  - Headache and Toothache
  - The Importance of the Hands and Feet
  - Motion Sickness and Nausea
  - Two Natural Tranquilizing Points

- Summary

- Good Luck, Good Health

- Massage At A Glance

ENHANCING MASSAGE THERAPY

The simple use of finger pressure on certain parts of the body can enhance the beneficial effects of massage. This is known as meridian therapy, or acupressure (acupuncture without the use of needles). When combined with the massage techniques you have already learned, this additional form of therapy can be very helpful indeed. You don't need to know a lot about acupressure to perform some of the basic procedures effectively.

Meridian therapy is an ancient and proven practice based on stimulating certain points of the body on the skin's surface. The aim is to promote wellness generally and, in some circumstances, to treat specific conditions (see next section).

The western world became interested in acupuncture in the mid-Seventies after President Nixon visited China and the Chinese government gave a demonstration of acupuncture techniques, which included surgery using acupuncture anesthesia instead of normal medical anesthesia. The demonstration generated tremendous interest, effectively introducing the therapy into western medicine.

At the time, we had several Japanese and Chinese medical doctors studying at our college. The college president, Dr Janse, recognized there were enormous therapeutic benefits in the practice of acupuncture. He immediately included a course on its theory and procedures in the final year of our studies. I believe this was the first such formal course introduced in the United States. Since then, acupuncture has grown enormously in popularity throughout the western world.

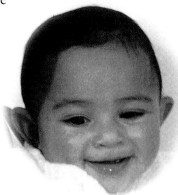

When I left college, I began applying the techniques we had studied, and saw how people responded to meridian therapy. I soon became convinced of the benefits to be achieved through a blend of therapies.

I have two good reasons for including this section in my book. First, I want to familiarize you with some of the meridian points. Second, I want to show you how, if used in tandem with your massage therapy, acupressure can add an extra dimension to your efforts. But first some background.

WHAT IS ACUPUNCTURE OR MERIDIAN THERAPY?

Meridian therapy has a long and impressive track record, the practice going back some 5,000 years. Ancient Egyptian, Persian, Indian and Chinese writings and inscriptions show that illnesses were treated using more than 1,000 acupuncture points located all over the body.

Oriental medicine theorizes that vital life force, or Qi (pronounced *chee*) courses through the body in specific channels called meridians. The meridians disperse their Qi in specific points just below the skin's surface, which are known as acupuncture points. There are 12 pairs of major meridians, 10 of which relate to organs of the body:

Lung	(LU)	Small intestine	(SI)
Large intestine	(LI)	Bladder	(BL)
Stomach	(ST)	Kidney	(KI)
Spleen	(SP)	Gall bladder	(GB)
Heart	(HT)	Liver	(LIV)
Pericardium	(P)	Tri-Heater	(TH)

There are also two unpaired meridians that run down the front and the back of the body in the midline:

Conception Vessel (CV) & Governing Vessel (GV)

It helps to think of the flow of Qi in the meridians as similar to blood flowing in our veins and arteries. Like blood, Qi is essential to the life of our tissues. Without it, tissue dies. A healthy person's Qi flows in a continuous and balanced manner. But illness or injury can cause too much or too little energy flow. This imbalance of Qi prompts tissue breakdown and disease.

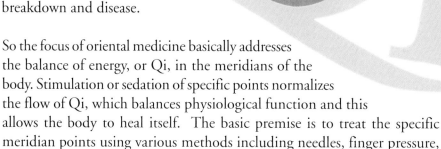

So the focus of oriental medicine basically addresses the balance of energy, or Qi, in the meridians of the body. Stimulation or sedation of specific points normalizes the flow of Qi, which balances physiological function and this allows the body to heal itself. The basic premise is to treat the specific meridian points using various methods including needles, finger pressure, and laser.

Acupuncture is the term most people are familiar with. The process specifically refers to the insertion of very fine needles into the acupuncture points. Hence the term, acu-puncture, or the 'accurate puncturing' of specific points.

I prefer the term *meridian therapy*, which includes any of the aforementioned methods.

Most modern acupuncturists use some 360 points. For our purposes we will discuss some of the more popular or effective meridian therapy points which can be used to enhance wellness, or as a first-aid approach to treat acute conditions.

Again, I wish to emphasize that the use of needles has no application in this book. Simple finger pressure on specific meridian points can be a very effective bonus to the massage techniques described earlier.

HOW DOES MERIDIAN THERAPY AFFECT THE BODY?

Among the many benefits of meridian therapy, perhaps the most important for children are those which have a direct and rather immediate effect on the balance of the central nervous system. Such stimulation:

- Balances brain and nervous system function.

- Releases morphine-like chemicals to combat painful conditions.

- Causes mental relaxation and produces a state of calmness and well-being.

- Enhances glandular function and hormonal balance.

- Improves the immune system.

- Boosts the body's repair and healing mechanism, thereby reducing excessive inflammation.

- Coordinates and balances muscle tone.

Ongoing research almost certainly means there will be further important advances made in meridian therapy. Meanwhile, there is nothing more rewarding than to see a young child improve rapidly before your eyes after only a few treatments.

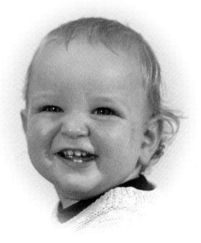

GETTING STARTED WITH ACUPRESSURE

Now that we have looked at the background, let's get started with some basic techniques.

First, we will highlight some of the important meridian points treated automatically when massaging the spine and back. Then we will familiarize ourselves with particular points you can target to achieve certain results or to treat specific illnesses and relieve common conditions.

I have found that teaching mothers about these basic points gives them a powerful tool to help their children recover their health naturally.

USING YOUR HANDS

It is easy to stimulate meridian points by gentle finger pressure (using either the thumb, forefinger or middle finger). Remember that acupuncture points are quite small and the application of the pad of your index finger will cover each point easily.

Sometimes, acupressure can be quite uncomfortable if an area is tender. So very gentle pressure is all you will ever need to apply to a baby. As with the massage techniques described earlier, the pressure you apply to your child should never be greater than that which you can comfortably withstand on your closed eyelid. In short, if you don't apply enough pressure to injure your eye, you certainly can't harm your child.

When treating several points, hold the pressure steadily on each point for 10-20 seconds. Sometimes, you may want to hold a single point for 30 seconds or more. Use a gentle, circular motion as you apply the pressure. Remember to watch your baby's face and follow your instincts. You will know when enough is enough, and if steady pressure is better than rhythmic massage on the point. It is generally considered to be better to under-treat than to over-treat. Sometimes, less is more.

WHAT IS THE BEST POSITION?

For treating the points along the spine, try lying on your back on a bed – or on the floor – and place your baby on top so you are both chest-to-chest.

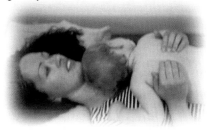

Your fingers will then fit perfectly on either side of the spine and you can apply gentle massaging pressure across the entire back area. If that feels comfortable and natural for you both, then the position is fine.

Some may feel it is more convenient to place the baby stomach down (prone) on a flat, safe surface like a change table or bench. The key is whether your baby is relaxed or not (many babies settle better when lying in the chest-to-chest position).

The acupuncture points on the front of the body are treated with the child lying comfortably face-up, while for those points on the hands and feet it doesn't matter whether the child is lying on its back or stomach. Remember to watch facial expressions to make sure the child is comfortable, adjusting positions as necessary.

POINTS, PROBLEMS AND SOLUTIONS

[1] The "All-In-One-Go" Approach

A series of very important acupressure points lie on the bladder meridian alongside the spine, approximately one finger's width to either side of the center. These are called Associated or Shu points and each corresponds to a specific organ. These are powerful points and their application can be a study in itself. Our pictures illustrate which points relate to different organs. The Bladder meridian is the largest meridian, starting at the corner of the eye, and ending with BL 67 (the Tsing point) at the side of the small toe (see page 113). By massaging the back, you cover the Associated (Shu) points, and many of the other Bladder meridian points.

We can simplify this very complex meridian by a few generalizations.

The upper back largely affects the organs in the chest itself, such as the heart and lungs. The middle back, between the shoulders, affects the stomach, liver and small intestines, and the lower back the bowel, bladder and kidneys. A child with stomach ache or colic, for example, relaxes very quickly when massaged in the area between the shoulders. Diarrhea or constipation responds well to lower back massage. A chest cold needs work in the upper back, just below the neck and between the shoulders.

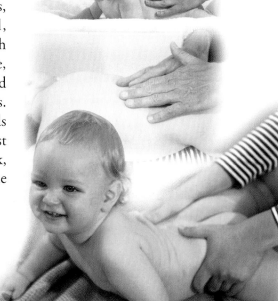

I would stress the importance of one particular Bladder point, BL 38, located in the area between the shoulders in the middle inner edge of the shoulder blade (on both sides). This is very good for stimulating energy and circulation in the head and chest. The Chinese name translates to "Rich for the Vitals", which means it has a very positive effect on the 'vital' organs. Use this point regularly, even if for only a quick rub during a busy day. Your child will love it.

BL 38

You can treat the entire series of Shu points by performing the following procedure.

C 7/T 1

With the baby lying chest to chest, simply place the fingers of both hands on each side of the little bumps in the center of the child's spine (the spinous processes). With your fingers now falling in line on either side of the spine, start at the base of the neck, between the shoulders, where we feel the first two prominent vertebrae (the spinous processes of C 7/T 1). Your fingers will then fall between the shoulder blades, and off to either side of the spinous processes. Begin a gentle kneading movement over this area of the spine for several minutes. Then move down to the next segment of the spine beginning immediately below and adjacent to the area you have just massaged. With a small baby you can cover the entire spine by moving the fingers down in two or three moves. A larger child may need a bit more. It is like painting a wall; make sure you cover each bit with at least one coat and don't miss any spots.

To cover the outer points on the Bladder Meridian (BL 36 - 49) just move your fingers out a bit further from the spine and repeat the process. Remember to include BL 38 so that you stimulate the organs in the chest!

By doing this you will have treated all of the Associated (Shu)points and many of the Bladder points, achieving a powerful stimulating and balancing effect on the various meridians of the body. You can work all the way down to the sacral bone, the bony area at the base of the spine (just above the coccyx or tailbone). Watch the child's face and assess the response. Most times the baby will relax into you and truly enjoy the procedure.

If the child is agitated then you may be pressing too hard, or you may have simply stimulated the area sufficiently. Move to the next part and return later to see if the problem is tenderness.

ACUPRESSURE POINTS

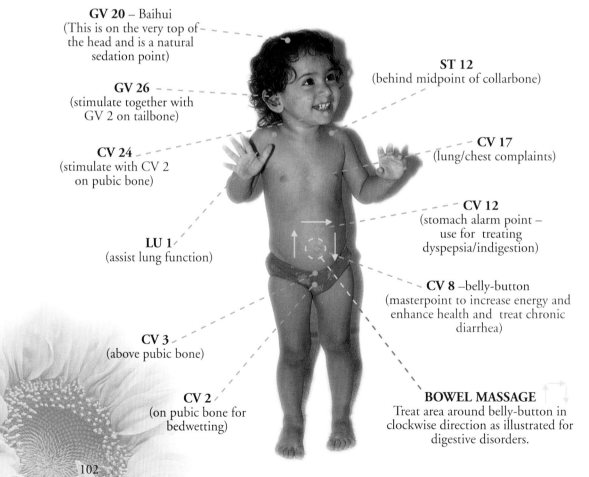

GV 20 – Baihui (This is on the very top of the head and is a natural sedation point)

GV 26 (stimulate together with GV 2 on tailbone)

CV 24 (stimulate with CV 2 on pubic bone)

LU 1 (assist lung function)

CV 3 (above pubic bone)

CV 2 (on pubic bone for bedwetting)

ST 12 (behind midpoint of collarbone)

CV 17 (lung/chest complaints)

CV 12 (stomach alarm point – use for treating dyspepsia/indigestion)

CV 8 –belly-button (masterpoint to increase energy and enhance health and treat chronic diarrhea)

BOWEL MASSAGE Treat area around belly-button in clockwise direction as illustrated for digestive disorders.

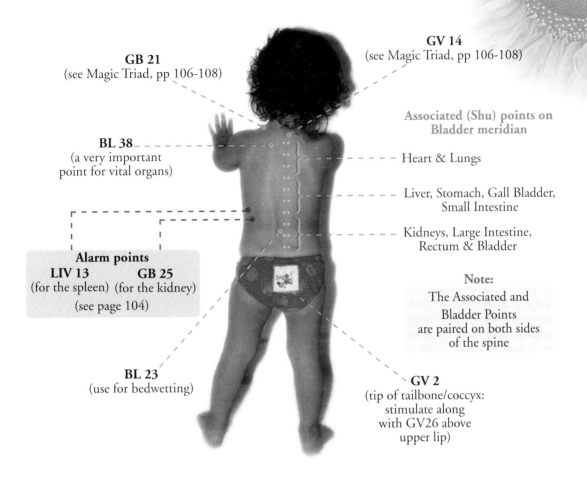

GB 21
(see Magic Triad, pp 106-108)

GV 14
(see Magic Triad, pp 106-108)

Associated (Shu) points on
Bladder meridian

BL 38
(a very important
point for vital organs)

Heart & Lungs

Liver, Stomach, Gall Bladder,
Small Intestine

Kidneys, Large Intestine,
Rectum & Bladder

Alarm points
LIV 13   **GB 25**
(for the spleen) (for the kidney)
(see page 104)

Note:
The Associated and
Bladder Points
are paired on both sides
of the spine

BL 23
(use for bedwetting)

GV 2
(tip of tailbone/coccyx:
stimulate along
with GV26 above
upper lip)

[2] Some Particularly Beneficial Points

As mentioned earlier, there are several points that may relate to certain common conditions in babies and small children. The list is long. But here are some specific points you may find helpful.

Lack of energy: Energy flows up the back and down the front of our body in a circular motion. Alteration of this normal energy flow can cause significant health problems. The single Conception Vessel (CV) meridian runs from below the lower lip down the front midline of the body to the area just in front of the anus. This channel, along with the posterior energy channel running up the back of the body, the Governing Vessel (GV), is one of the master energy channels of the body. By treating these meridians you can improve and restore energy balance. (See illustrations on pages 102 & 103.)

To stimulate the Conception Vessel (in the front) simultaneously rub CV 24, the point directly below the lower lip and, CV 2, on the pubic bone, for about 20-30 seconds. Next treat the Governing Vessel by simultaneously rubbing the point above the upper lip, GV 26, and GV 2, on the tip of the tailbone (coccyx) for 20-30 seconds. This technique helps improve coordination and is used to alleviate learning difficulties. You can do this once a day for several days at a time, and then whenever you notice the child becoming irritable or restless.

ALARM POINTS

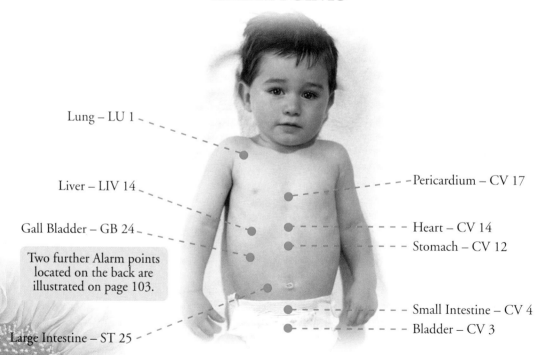

Lung – LU 1

Liver – LIV 14

Gall Bladder – GB 24

Two further Alarm points located on the back are illustrated on page 103.

Large Intestine – ST 25

Pericardium – CV 17

Heart – CV 14
Stomach – CV 12

Small Intestine – CV 4
Bladder – CV 3

A word on Alarm points: Each meridian has an Alarm point which acts as an early warning system to indicate if there is an imbalance in that meridian. An Alarm point often can be tender to touch if there is a problem. You can also use Alarm points with good effect to treat a meridian. Look at the Alarm point illustration (page 104) if your child has any specific illness and see if there is tenderness in the Alarm point that associates with the organ affected. For example, in acute bronchitis, check for tenderness of LU 1. You can treat an Alarm point with simple massage even if it isn't tender.

Bed-wetting: Immediately above the pubic bone is the second point on the Conception Vessel, or CV 2. The Alarm point for the Bladder meridian, CV 3, lies an inch or so above this, approximately two inches above the pubic bone.

Pressure exerted on these two points is often used to treat enuresis, or bedwetting. You can also treat BL 23 by massaging the lower lumbar region. It may be handy to know these as your child grows up, because bed-wetting is a very common and disturbing problem.

Chronic diarrhea: Located in the middle of the belly button (umbilicus) is the meridian point CV8 (known to the Chinese as the 'Shrine of God'). The Chinese believe energy enters the body at this point at birth, and leaves it at death. The point may be treated either by finger pressure or laser acupuncture. It is viewed as a Master point and is checked and treated regularly for many childhood diseases. It is especially helpful in relieving chronic diarrhea and tension.

Digestive disorders: People with digestive ailments are often extremely tender in the deeper tissues around the umbilicus. Using your first two fingers and gently massaging this area can make the whole body feel better. Just treating the area around the umbilicus within a five-centimeter radius will work wonders for digestion and elimination.

Tummy upsets: Midway between the umbilicus and the bony point where the sternum ends is CV 12, the Alarm point for the stomach. Children (and adults) are usually tender in this area when they have tummy upsets. By gently rubbing this point, you can ease symptoms including dyspepsia, nausea, colic and vomiting. This point can be carefully treated even when there is considerable discomfort in the abdomen.

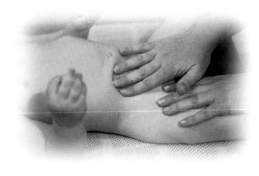

(3) James and the Magic Triad

James was an unwell six-year-old. He suffered variously from allergies, digestive problems and symptoms suggestive of attention deficit disorder (ADD). Altogether he was not happy. Neither were his parents. They had taken him to a number of health care practitioners and specialists, but his general condition had improved only slightly. They felt powerless being unable to help when their young son was so continually distressed.

They discussed James' problems with me and I suggested they perform acupressure on a group of meridian points – actually five in number – known as the 'Magic Triad.'

Treatment of these points can induce a feeling of well-being and significantly improve health. The Magic Triad consists of two points on the left shoulder and two corresponding points on the right plus the fifth point located in the upper region of the back. There is a point called Stomach 12 (ST12) on each shoulder, and, likewise, a point on each shoulder called Bladder 21 (BL 21). The fifth point, located centrally in the upper region of the back, is called Governing Vessel 14 (GV 14).

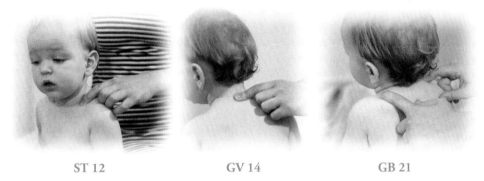

| ST 12 | GV 14 | GB 21 |

These are clearly indicated in the accompanying photographs, but it is a good idea to find them physically on yourself first before you treat your child. Some of the points are tender in an adult and you will get a better feel for their precise location this way.

To find ST 12, place your fingers into the area on the top of one of your shoulders right behind the collarbone. Then hook your fingers onto the back of the collarbone midway along its length, where you will find a central, sensitive point. This is ST 12, which connects internally to, and has a powerful influence on, eight other meridians of the body. Do the same to find the corresponding ST 12 point on the other shoulder.

Next find GV 14 (between the spinous processes of the first two prominent vertebrae at the base of your neck, immediately between your shoulders). Then, finally, go to the top of the trapezius muscle, midway between the neck and the tip of the shoulder, and palpate around until you find a tense and probably tender point. This is GB 21. Once again, do the same to find the corresponding GB 21 point on the other shoulder.

By stimulating these five points you help create a healthy balance for the entire body. The immune system gets a gentle boost and a general sense of well-being follows. When a child or grown-up is unwell, I recommend you treat these points twice a day with light finger pressure over the area. You can do both sides at once, working each point for up to a minute.

Why do we always feel so good when someone comes up behind us and rubs our shoulders, kneading our trapezius muscles between their thumbs and forefingers? It has a lot to do with the fact that these points are being stimulated in the process.

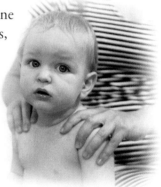

CASE HISTORY: I showed James' parents how to work on the Magic Triad, just as I had been taught by my instructor years before. They went away and began treating the young boy twice a day, for just several minutes each time. James picked up quickly after each episode. He became brighter, his face always lighting up when they gently massaged these points morning and night.

Perhaps, best of all, his parents became involved in James' healing. The three of them became as one in the battle to regain his health. It was rewarding to watch his father take part in the process. He was no longer the helpless parent, and he gained real pride knowing he could do something to help his son back to a state of wellness.

Sometimes, healing your child goes beyond the immediate task. It can also help relationships and restore self-esteem.

[4] Lung Problems: Asthma and Upper Respiratory Tract Infections

Meridian therapy can help relieve respiratory conditions, such as asthma, bronchitis or croup. It is important to understand I am not suggesting that a parent stop medicating a child who has asthma, which can be very serious and often requires medical help.

However, there are many instances when parents can help a child by performing a simple, safe procedure that brings relief and speeds the entire healing process.

In such circumstances check and treat the Lung Alarm point (LU 1) on the outer part of the front of the chest, just beneath the collarbone. There will be a tense and tender point in the area of the pectoralis minor muscle and this relates to the first point on the Lung meridian. Gentle digital pressure of this area can significantly help lung function.

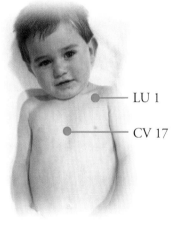

LU 1

CV 17

Similarly, gentle pressure on the area around and including the 'big bump' (GV 14) at the base of the neck can alleviate lung problems. And remember to include the other important point (CV 17), which is on the breastbone level with the nipples.

There are two further Lung meridian points with which I would like you to become familiar. If you bend your elbow slightly you will notice the crease there. Feeling the forearm musculature in the outer part of this crease you will find a sensitive point which relates to the 5th point on the Lung meridian (LU 5). That is the first.

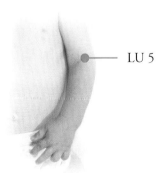

LU 5

The second is Lung 7 (LU 7) which is on the thumb side of the forearm, about three of your child's fingerbreadths up from the thumb base. It is located on the palmar side of the forearm, about where you would feel your pulse. Both these points can be used to treat problems like upper respiratory infections and asthma.

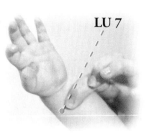

LU 7

CASE HISTORY: Many children with chronic asthma will melt into your arms when you stimulate the points described in this section. I remember the experience of young Zach, who had chronic asthma that saw him rushed to hospital on many occasions late at night.

He would spend a day or two on a nebulizer and then weeks on medication. His attacks occurred regularly. His wheezing worsened with cold weather and his mother would fret about whether this would be another night spent at the hospital.

So I showed Zach's parents how to use acupressure, first working on the Associated points between the shoulder blades in the upper dorsal spine immediately below the neck. His mother would pay particular attention to the area around the second and third dorsal vertebrae, the Associated points for the lungs. Interestingly, Zach would flinch the first few times she rubbed this area. He would relax after three or four minutes of rubbing, and then breathe easier. His parents could hear the wheezing ease as he let go!

They would then massage the CV 17 point on his sternum.

While Zach's problems didn't disappear altogether, his parents now at least had a tool that enabled them to influence his condition in a very positive way. They could at last give their son relief instead of panicking at the first sign of a wheeze and rushing him off to hospital.

Keep in mind, at all times, that asthma can be very serious and even life-threatening. If the child is in distress then seek immediate medical help. Treating these points in the meantime can be most helpful.

[5]   Headache and Toothache

Many children experience toothache at an early age, one of the painful "teething" problems of growing up. Equally, they may also have headaches. Both painful conditions can be relieved dramatically by massaging the web of the thumb, deep in the muscle belly between the thumb and forefinger.

This area, often quite tender when exposed to pressure, is the fourth point on the Large Intestine meridian (LI 4, called Hegu, or Hoku in Chinese). Refer to Tsing points on the hands on page 113.

For children with toothache, you may also apply an ice cube for one to five minutes, but be careful not to leave the ice continually for more than two to three minutes without rubbing the area so that you don't freeze the skin.

The use of ice on children (and adults) was endorsed several years ago by a leading dental group that recommended this course to parents, particularly for children sensitive to medication. Personally, I would suggest using it as a first line of defense simply because it is natural! The endorphins released by the body are estimated to be up to100 times more powerful than morphine, and simple stimulation of LI 4 causes the release of endorphins. The pharmacy between your ears knows exactly how much endorphin needs to be released to ease the pain!

CASE HISTORY: Martin was having a lot of trouble getting his first teeth. Nothing seemed to relieve his discomfort. He cried for hours on end and his parents were quite sleep-deprived. His mother was taught to massage gently the thumb web on both sides, morning, afternoon and night, and whenever she felt it necessary. She was amazed at how effectively it worked! Martin would calm down in 10 minutes and fall back to sleep, whereas before he would cry for hours.

I have seen this work for toothache as well as all kinds of headaches. Massaging LI 4 will also help ease the overall muscle and joint aches associated with flu and colds.

ANOTHER TIP: Pressure on the second toe (the 45th point at the end of the Stomach meridian) often will bring dramatic relief for headaches.

[6] The Importance of the Hands and Feet

If I had a choice of one place to massage, given time limitations and perhaps a restless child, I would start with the hands and/or feet. It takes about 10 minutes and the entire body benefits.

Simply massage each finger, working from fingertips to the knuckles, concentrating on the area around the fingernail and fingertip. Work the thumb web gently because it can be tender. (The tenderness usually occurs later in life as we accumulate toxins and stresses in our bodies with aging). Then work the palm to the wrist.

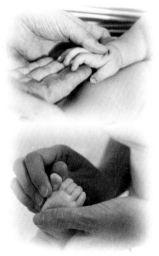

The same applies to the foot, working each toe and then the entire foot.

In acupuncture theory all meridians, or energy channels of the body, either begin or end on the hands and feet (except for the Conception and Governing Vessels). Indeed, there is a branch of Korean acupuncture that specifically focuses on the hands for treating the entire body.

HAND TSING POINTS

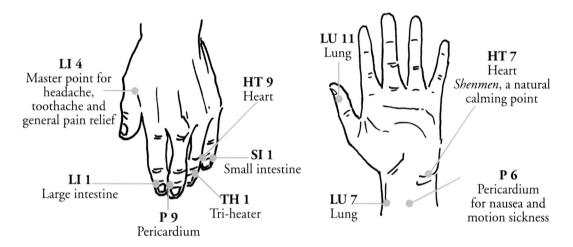

LI 4
Master point for headache, toothache and general pain relief

HT 9
Heart

SI 1
Small intestine

LI 1
Large intestine

TH 1
Tri-heater

P 9
Pericardium

LU 11
Lung

HT 7
Heart
Shenmen, a natural calming point

P 6
Pericardium for nausea and motion sickness

LU 7
Lung

FOOT TSING POINTS

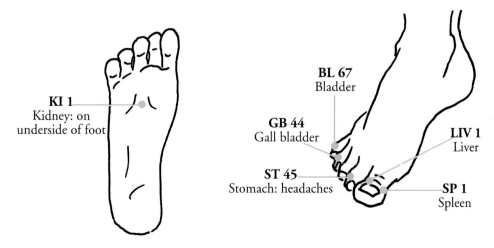

KI 1
Kidney: on underside of foot

BL 67
Bladder

GB 44
Gall bladder

LIV 1
Liver

ST 45
Stomach: headaches

SP 1
Spleen

The Tsing, or "Beginning and End" Points

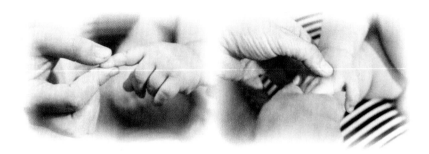

The Tsing points are also known as the "Beginning and End" points of the upper and lower body meridians and are located a "rice grain" width to the side of the nail bed. Working the tip of the fingers therefore stimulates the Tsing points and affects all the meridians of the upper body.

The same concept applies to the toes. Working the general nail bed area will stimulate the Tsing points of the lower body meridians. Overall massage in these areas will bring good results.

CASE HISTORY: Little Jonathon was having a very hard time with recurring upper respiratory tract infections. His mother was taught hand and foot massage, and he immediately loved the procedure! In a short time, the frequency and intensity of infections reduced dramatically. His mother certainly knew that stimulating his hands and feet helped his body function better, and she continues to this day to perform regular massage on Jonathon. Her only complaint is now he is 14 and asks: "What about my foot massage?!" She is trying to arrange a reciprocal agreement.

ANOTHER TIP: Some babies will wake up if you try massaging their feet when they are asleep. We know the sole of the foot is the most ticklish part of the body on most people. However, many babies will actually fall asleep while their hands and feet are being massaged.

[7] Motion Sickness and Nausea

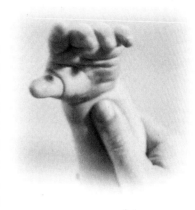

Many people who suffer from motion sickness know that stimulation of a small point (Pericardium or P 6) on the fleshy underside of the wrists, about three finger widths up from the wrist crease directly in the midline, eases nausea and motion sickness. (Use the finger width of the patient, not yours). Try this with a child who has a gastric upset, or travel sickness.

[8] Two Natural Tranquilizing Points

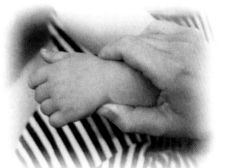

Shenmen is a point used to treat insomnia, worry, anxiety, heart palpitations and various mental disorders. A child who is agitated for whatever reason will often respond nicely to pressure on this point on the underside of the wrist.

Shenmen (which means 'The Door to Heaven') is the seventh point (H 7) on the Heart meridian. It is located on the little finger side on the wrist crease. Its name derives from the effect it has of calming the mind and opening the door to sleep. What a handy point for a parent to know! I have seen Shenmen work time and time again on distressed children.

CASE HISTORY: Susan was barely 12 months old and just plain irritable. Months of stress through lack of sleep had created an habitual, broken sleep pattern. Her parents had had enough, and so had she. Her mother started rubbing the Shenmen point, using simple finger pressure. After several nights, the baby calmed down and began sleeping better. Her mother also noted that Susan would look up at her as she gently massaged her wrists (one at a time). The baby would visibly begin to breathe more easily as she slipped quietly towards sleep.

ANOTHER TIP: You may find that treating one side is enough. Use both sides if you need to give an extra 'dose'. Watch as 'the Door to Heaven' begins to open under your loving touch.

Baihui (pronounced *bay-way*) is the point of choice for tranquilizing and sedation. It is almost always used for treating psychiatric disorders, or in any disease where there is a psychogenic component. In other words, when you have any agitation or anxiety, you treat this point.

Positioned in the center on the very top of our heads, it is the 20th point on the Governing Vessel (GV 20). **Baihui**, (in the middle of the scalp and in line with the ears) translates as the '*meeting point of 100 diseases*'. Treating this point confronts many disease processes.

For our purposes, we will concentrate on the soothing effect of treating GV 20, which may explain why it feels so good to have the top of your head rubbed! This point is there to be used whenever we have a child that is agitated or distressed. As you gently rub the top of the child's head, strategically place one finger over the point and rub it specifically for several minutes. Sedation is soothing, so your technique should match the effect you are trying to create.

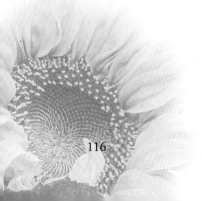

SUMMARY

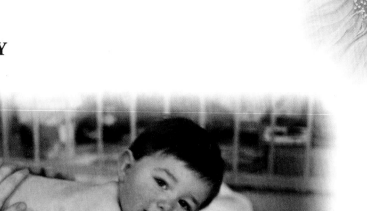

Remember that by massaging your child you are stimulating acupressure points all the time. When you massage the back, you automatically affect the Associated points and the Bladder meridian. When doing the hands and feet you cover all the meridians. You simply have to watch your child's reaction to see if he or she has had enough. If the child is enjoying it, continue. If agitated, then it is either time to stop, or try another approach (such as moving to another part of the body or changing the pressure).

By including some of the points mentioned you can make your massage session even more effective. You don't have to memorize these points. Refer to this book when there is a certain condition you feel may need special attention. Knowing that the points exist simply enables you to approach your child with the intent of balancing the body's energy. It also makes you realize that, each time, your caring touch stimulates your child's innate healing mechanism. It is wonderful to know you can achieve such positive results merely by using your hands.

GOOD LUCK, GOOD HEALTH!

I am always amazed when I watch my tiny patients and see how they lock their eyes onto mine. It is a magical feeling when their little hands grasp out and touch me as I work on them. I imagine each glance and touch sending millions of impulses to their amazing brains, putting down new neural connections and pathways, reinforcing their reflexes and knowledge of the world.

By massaging our children, we help stimulate the development of their nervous system. We enhance a positive body image so that they grow into adults with good self-esteem and appreciation of who they are. They know they are special because they have been nurtured and touched in a loving way since their first days on this planet.

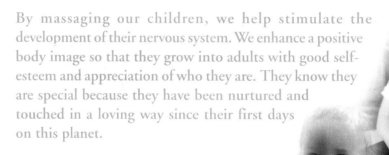

I hope that you incorporate these techniques in a system that works for you and your child. Remember it takes time to develop any skill, and at first you may feel awkward and even clumsy. Don't worry, just get on your bike and go for it.

Watch your baby's face as he or she delights in the wonderful sensations that occur during the application of therapeutic massage. You will improve the health of your child, your family and even yourself by applying your newfound skills.

Good luck and good health!

MASSAGE AT A GLANCE

The following is a handy guide to the massage techniques we have covered in this book. I suggest you photo-copy it, cover it in plastic, and use it as you massage your child.

After applying these procedures a few times, you will more than likely develop your own style and sequence based around what is comfortable for you and your baby. That's fine.

Lying Face-Down: the Prone Position

Stage One: The Head and Spine
Massage the following areas:

- From the top of head backwards to the base of the skull
- Upper neck/base of skull to trapezius muscles and tips of shoulders
- Between shoulders headwards to trapezius muscles and tips of shoulders
- Trapezius muscles and shoulder joints
- Lower back sweeping upwards to base of neck and outwards to tips of shoulders
- Sweep the sacrum outwards over buttocks and hips
- Finish with light stroking downwards from neck to buttocks

Stage Two: The Back of the Lower Extremities
Massage the following areas:

- Sweep upwards from the heel to the back of knees
- Massage the back of the knees
- Sweep up the back of the thigh from behind the knee onto and over the buttocks
- Return to foot and massage ankle, and then ball of foot to the heel
- Massage the toes

Lying Face up - The Supine Position

Stage Three: Face, Head and Neck:
Massaging the following while standing at
the head of your baby:

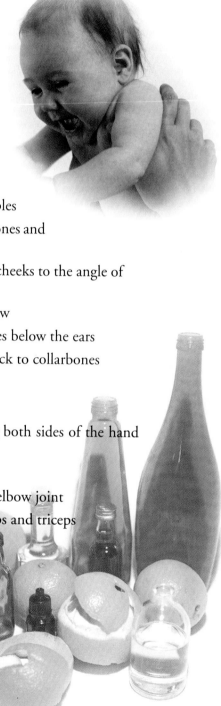

- Cradle the head/face using the 'prayer hold'
- Sweep outwards from top/center of head outwards to the ears
- Massage temples in a circular motion
- Sweep the center of forehead out to the temples
- Sweep out from under the eyes to the cheekbones and ears
- Sweep out over the upper lip area across the cheeks to the angle of the jaw
- Sweep outwards from lower lip to angle of jaw
- Sweep outward from under the chin to tissues below the ears
- Sweep out from under jaw, down front of neck to collarbones

Stage Four: Arms and Hands:

- Massage from finger tips to the wrist, doing both sides of the hand simultaneously
- Sweep from wrist to elbow
- Perform circular massage to the front of the elbow joint
- Sweep from elbow to shoulder, treating biceps and triceps
- Use the 'O' grip from wrist to shoulder

Stage Five: Chest and Abdomen:

- Sweep from center of chest out to sides of thorax (follow downward slope of ribs)
- Massage area of diaphragm where abdominal muscles attach to lower ribs
- Circular area around umbilicus
- Colon sweep, from lower right quadrant (area of appendix) upwards to right shoulder, stopping where ribs end, from right to left across the transverse colon, just below ribs from upper left quadrant down to lower left quadrant above groin
- Gentle sweep around genital area

Stage Six: Front of Lower Extremities:

- Sweep up the front of the leg from ankle to knee
- Sweep up the thigh from the knee to the hip
- Sweep up the outer side of the thigh from knee to hip
- Return to foot and sweep the top of the foot from the toes to the ankle
- Massage each toe, pulling gently and then bending back
- Bend entire foot back, stretching ball of foot and calf

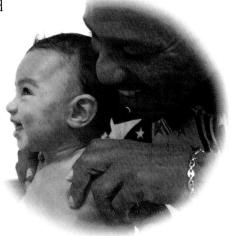

BIBLIOGRAPHY

- Ackerman, Diane, A Natural History of the Senses, New York, Vintage Books, (1995).

- Amaro, Dr. J., International Academy of Clinical Acupuncture, (1991).

- Brennan, Paula, Transactional analyst, Personal correspondence, Perth, Western Australia (1998).

- Bryner, Dr. P., Chiropractor and researcher, Personal correspondence, Perth, Western Australia (1999).

- Chopra, Dr. Deepak, Unconditional Life. New York, Bantam, (1991)

- Erickson, Milton H., various works.

- Goldberg, Stephen, MD, Clinical Neuroanatomy Made Ridiculously Simple, Miami, Fla., Medmaster, Inc., (1986).

- Janse, Joseph. Principles and Practice of Chiropractic, National College of Chiropractic, (1976).

- Jenkins, David B., Hollinshead, W. Henry, Biblis, M (Editor), Hollinshead's Functional Anatomy of the Limbs and Back, W. B. Saunders and Co., (1998).

- Life Magazine, (August 1997).

- Netter, Frank H., Nervous System, The Ciba Collection of Medical Illustrations, (1962).

- Pearce, Joseph Chilton. The Crack in the Cosmic Egg (New York, Crown, 1988).

- Touch Research Institute, Various research articles, University of Miami School of Medicine, Miami, Florida. (1998).

NOTES

NOTES

NOTES

NOTES